Instructor's Manual
for the
Laboratory Manual

Concepts of
HUMAN
ANATOMY & physiology

fourth edition

Kent M. Van De Graaff
University of Utah
Stuart Ira Fox
Pierce College

Prepared by
Jeffrey and Karianne Prince

WCB Wm. C. Brown Publishers
Dubuque, IA Bogota Boston Buenos Aires Caracas Chicago
Guilford, CT London Madrid Mexico City Sydney Toronto

A Times Mirror Company

ISBN 0-697-16080-7

Printed in the United States of America by Wm. C. Brown Communications, Inc., 2460 Kerper Boulevard, Dubuque, Iowa, 52001

10 9 8 7 6 5 4 3 2 1

Contents

Preface

The laboratory is a good place to teach anatomy and physiology. Students can interact with one another and with an instructor in small groups, and a relatively large amount of time can be devoted to relatively small chunks of information based on the laboratory exercises. In order for this valuable time to be used most effectively, the laboratory exercises should reinforce and complement lecture material and be perceived by students as important, not simply as busy work.

The *Laboratory Manual for Concepts of Human Anatomy and Physiology* helps instructors to achieve these goals. A wide variety of exercises is presented so that an instructor can select an exercise that reinforces almost any topic covered at a given time in lecture. Students are encouraged to use their textbook, *Concepts of Human Anatomy and Physiology*, 4th ed., before, during, and following each exercise. The pertinence of each exercise to the lecture portion of the course is thus firmly established.

This *Instructor's Manual* contains information needed to successfully teach an anatomy and physiology laboratory course using the *Laboratory Manual for Concepts of Human Anatomy and Physiology*. The exercise overviews contain a concise introduction explaining the purpose of the exercise, a list of needed materials, and answers to any labeling or table exercise presented in the laboratory exercise. These overviews should provide all of the information needed to prepare for each laboratory exercise. Answers for all laboratory reports are contained in a separate section. Appendices in the *Instructor's Manual* include a list of biological supply houses (supplementing the list presented in the *Laboratory Manual for Concepts of Human Anatomy and Physiology*), recipes for commonly made solutions, and tips for dissection.

We sincerely appreciate Dr. Kent M. Van De Graaff for his encouragement and assistance during the writing of this *Instructor's Manual*. We also appreciate the faculty of the Zoology Department at Brigham Young University for their support during this project.

Correlation of Laboratory and Lecture

Textbook Chapter	Laboratory Exercise	Laboratory Exercise Title
1	1	Body Organization and Terminology
	2	Microscope and Metric System
	3	Homeostasis and Negative Feedback
2	4	Measurement of Plasma Glucose, Protein, and Cholesterol
3	5	Cell Structure and Cell Division
3,4	6	Genetic Control of Metabolism
5	7	Diffusion, Osmosis, and Tonicity
6	8	Histology
7	9	The Integumentary System
8	10	Structure of Bone Tissue
9	11	Skeletal System: The Axial Skeleton
10	12	Skeletal System: The Appendicular Skeleton
11	13	Articulations
12	14	Neural Control of Skeletal Muscle Contraction
	15	Summation, Tetanus, and Fatigue
13	16	Muscles of the Head and Neck
	17	Muscles of the Pectoral Girdle and Upper Extremity
	18	Muscles of the Trunk and Lower Extremity
	19	Cat Musculature
15,16	20	Brain and Cranial Nerves
16,18	21	Spinal Cord, Spinal Nerves, and Spinal Reflexes
18	22	Cutaneous Receptors
	23	Eyes and Vision
	24	Ears and Hearing
	25	Taste
19	26	Endocrine System
20,24	27	Red Blood Cells and Oxygen Transport
20,23	28	Total and Differential White Blood Cell Counts
20,30	29	Blood Types
20,21	30	Heart and Arteries
21,23	31	Veins, Lymphatics, and Fetal Circulation
21	32	Effects of Drugs on the Frog Heart
	33	Electrocardiogram
	34	Mean Electrical Axis of the Ventricles
21,22	35	Heart Sounds and Measurement of Blood Pressure
22	36	Cardiovascular System and Physical Fitness
24	37	Respiratory System
	38	Measurements of Pulmonary Function
	39	Effects of Exercise on the Respiratory System
25	40	Urinary System
	41	Renal Regulation of Fluid and Electrolyte Balance
	42	Renal Plasma Clearance of Urea
	43	Clinical Examination of the Urine

Exercise Overviews

Exercise 1 Body Organization and Terminology

INTRODUCTION

Anatomy is a descriptive science. This laboratory exercise is designed to introduce students to body organization and terminology. Students need to understand proper terminology to understand anatomy. This exercise also discusses levels of organization, such as cells, tissues, organs, and systems.

MATERIALS

1. Anatomical charts and illustrations
2. Human torso model
3. Reference text
4. Colored pencils

KEY TO LABELING EXERCISES

Figure 1.1 Major body regions and localized areas.

1. Cervical region
2. Deltoid region
3. Axillary region
4. Brachium
5. Elbow
6. Lumbar region
7. Antebrachium
8. Buttock
9. Thigh
10. Popliteal fossa
11. Calf
12. Plantar surface
13. Upper extremity
14. Lower extremity
15. Head
16. Neck
17. Thorax
18. Cubital fossa
19. Abdomen
20. Pubic region
21. Palmar surface
22. Patellar region

Figure 1.2 An anterior view of body cavities.

1. Pleural cavity
2. Pericardial cavity
3. Diaphragm
4. Abdominal cavity
5. Pelvic cavity
6. Thoracic cavity
7. Abdominopelvic cavity

Figure 1.3 A medial view of body cavities.

1. Thoracic cavity
2. Diaphragm
3. Abdominal cavity
4. Pelvic cavity
5. Brain
6. Cranial cavity
7. Vertebral canal
8. Spinal cord
9. Anterior cavity
10. Posterior cavity

Exercise 2 Microscope and Metric System

INTRODUCTION

This laboratory exercise is designed to introduce students to the microscope. Many scientific discoveries were possible only through the microscope. An understanding of the use of a microscope is necessary so that the student will be able to examine the microscopic anatomy of the organs later in the course. Students are also introduced to the metric system, which is the universal measurement system in science. A working knowledge of the metric system is necessary so that students will be able to make measurements and calculations in this laboratory.

MATERIALS

1. Compound microscope
2. Prepared microscope slides (with the letter *e*)
3. Lens paper

Exercise 3 Homeostasis and Negative Feedback

INTRODUCTION

This exercise introduces students to negative feedback, in regulating both temperature and pulse. Negative feedback is a concept that appears often in physiology but can be hard to understand, so this exercise is appropriate to illustrate these concepts.

MATERIALS

1. Watch or clock with a second hand
2. Constant-temperature water bath

Exercise 4 Measurement of Plasma Glucose, Protein, and Cholesterol

INTRODUCTION

Three molecules found in the blood are glucose, protein, and cholesterol. These molecules have very important physiological roles, and so they are carefully regulated. This exercise introduces students to measurement techniques using a colorimeter so they can measure the levels of these molecules in plasma. It is important to remember that the colorimeter must be zeroed using a blank for each of the different measuring methods. Standard curves must also be made in order to measure the concentration of the serum if it is taken from dogs or cats.

MATERIALS

1. Test tubes, mechanical pipettors, microliter pipettes (40 μl, 50 μl, and 100 μl capacities)
2. Constant-temperature water bath, set at 37°C
3. Colorimeter and cuvettes
4. Cholesterol kit (Medical Analysis Systems, Inc., available from Curtin-Matheson Scientific, Inc.)
5. Protein human albumin standards (purchased or previously diluted) of the following concentrations: 2,4,6,8,10 g/dl
6. Glucose kit ("glucose liquicolor" from Stanbio, available from Curtin-Matheson Scientific, Inc.)
7. Biuret reagent: add 45 g of sodium potassium tartarate and 15 g of $CuSO_4$–$5H_2O$ to a 1.0-liter volumetric flask; fill three-quarters full with 0.2 N NaOH; shake to dissolve; add 5.0 g of potassium iodide, and fill to volume with 0.2 N NaOH
8. Artificial serum with known values (available from supply houses), or serum from dogs or cats (available from veterinarians)

Exercise 5 Cell Structure and Cell Division

INTRODUCTION

This exercise is designed to introduce students to the structures and functions of a cell. Emphasis is placed on learning the organelles and their cellular function. Understanding cell structure and function is essential to understanding the principles of anatomy and physiology. Electron micrographs can be used effectively to illustrate the different organelles of the cell. This exercise could be combined with exercise 8.

MATERIALS

1. Compound microscope
2. Prepared slides of whitefish blastula
3. Lens paper
4. Reference text
5. Colored pencils

KEY TO LABELING EXERCISES

Figure 5.1 The cell.

1. Microtubules
2. Mitochondria
3. Cell membrane
4. Endoplasmic reticulum
5. Lysosome
6. Nucleus
7. Nucleolus
8. Chromatin
9. Golgi apparatus
10. Vacuole
11. Centriole
12. Cytoplasm
13. Ribosomes

Figure 5.2 The sequence of mitosis.

1. Centrioles
2. Nucleus
3. Interphase
4. Centromeres
5. Prophase
6. Spindle fibers
7. Metaphase
8. Anaphase
9. Telophase
10. Daughter cells

Figure 5.3 The process of meiosis.

1. Prophase I
2. Metaphase I
3. Anaphase I
4. Telophase I
5. Daughter cells
6. Prophase II
7. Metaphase II
8. Anaphase II
9. Telophase II
10. Daughter cells

Exercise 6 Genetic Control of Metabolism

INTRODUCTION

This exercise is designed to introduce students to gene regulation of metabolism. Phenylketonuria and alkaptonuria are diseases caused by defective genes, and in this exercise, students will measure the quantities of phenylpyruvic acid and homogentisic acid. (Silver nitrate must be stored in brown bottles in order to maintain its reactivity.)

MATERIALS

1. Test tubes, Pasteur pipettes (droppers), urine collection cups
2. Urine samples
3. Phenistix (Ames), silver nitrate (3 g/dl), 10% ammonium hydroxide, 40% sodium hydroxide

Exercise 7 Diffusion, Osmosis, and Tonicity

INTRODUCTION

This exercise is designed to introduce students to osmosis. Students will first experiment with a thistle tube to see the movement of water caused by osmosis. Then students will place red blood cells in solutions of different tonicity to see the effects of osmolality on red blood cells. Cells placed in a hypertonic solution will crenate, and cells placed in a hypotonic solution will swell and eventually lyse.

MATERIALS

1. Test tubes, thistle tubes, dialysis tubing
2. Beakers, ring stands, burette clamps
3. Lancets, alcohol swabs
4. Microscopes, slides, cover slips, and Pasteur pipettes (droppers)
5. Sucrose (30 g/dl) and sodium chloride solutions (0.20 g, 0.45 g, 0.85 g, 3.5 g, and 10 g per dl each)

Exercise 8 Histology

INTRODUCTION

This exercise is designed to introduce students to the four primary tissue types. Functions of these different tissue types, as well as where these tissues are located, should be emphasized to help the student understand the functions of the organs to be studied later. This exercise could be combined with exercise 5 in one laboratory period.

MATERIALS

1. Microscopes and lens paper
2. Prepared slides of the different tissues to be observed
3. Histology atlas
4. Colored pencils

KEY TO LABELING EXERCISES

Figure 8.1 Epithelial tissues.

1. Columnar epithelium
2. Simple squamous epithelium
3. Stratified squamous epithelium
4. Ciliated columnar epithelium
5. Cuboidal epithelium
6. Transitional epithelium
7. Pseudostratified columnar epithelium

Figure 8.2 Mesenchymal tissue.

1. Mesenchymal cell
2. Homogenous matrix

Figure 8.3 Connective tissue proper.

1. Loose connective tissue
2. Adipose connective tissue
3. Reticular connective tissue
4. Dense fibrous connective tissue
5. Elastic connective tissue

Figure 8.4 Cartilage tissue.

a. Hyaline cartilage
   1. Lacunae
   2. Chondrocyte

b. Fibrocartilage
   3. Lacuna
   4. Collagenous bundles

c. Elastic cartilage
   5. Chondrocyte
   6. Elastic fibers

Figure 8.5 Bone tissue.
1. Lamella
2. Central canal
3. Canaliculi
4. Lamella
5. Osteocyte within a lacuna

Figure 8.6 Vascular tissue.
1. Erythrocytes
2. Thrombocytes
3. Basophil
4. Neutrophil
5. Eosinophil
6. Lymphocyte
7. Monocyte

Figure 8.7 Muscular tissue.
a. Smooth muscle tissue
  1. Nucleus

b. Cardiac muscle tissue
  2. Intercalated disc
  3. Nucleus

c. Skeletal muscle tissue
  4. Nucleus
  5. Striation

Figure 8.8 Nervous tissue.
a. Neuroglial cells
b. Neuron
  1. Dendrites
  2. Cell body
  3. Nucleus
  4. Axon
  5. Schwann cell neurolemmocyte
  6. Branches of axon

Exercise 9 The Integumentary System

INTRODUCTION

This exercise is designed to introduce students to the integumentary system. Students examine the microscopic structure of the skin, and they prepare ink prints to look at dermal patterns. They are also introduced to the associated structures of the integumentary system as well as the layers of the skin.

MATERIALS

1. Microscope
2. Prepared slides of human skin (showing hair and associated glands) and a longitudinal section of fingertip
3. Magnifying glass
4. Reference text
5. Drawing pencils and colored pencils
6. Ink pad and black ink (washable)

KEY TO LABELING EXERCISES

Figure 9.1 A section of skin.
1. Stratum corneum
2. Stratum lucidum
3. Stratum granulosum
4. Stratum spinosum
5. Stratum basale
6. Papillary layer
7. Reticular layer
8. Epidermis
9. Dermis
10. Hypodermis

Figure 9.2 A diagram of a hair, a hair follicle, a sebaceous gland, and an arrector pili muscle.
1. Epidermis
2. Follicle
3. Shaft
4. Duct of sebaceous gland
5. Sebaceous gland
6. Arrector pili muscle
7. Root
8. Internal root sheath
9. External root sheath
10. Bulb
11. Dermal papilla
12. Root sheath

Figure 9.3 Photomicrograph of a fingernail of a human neonate.

1. Matrix
2. Nail root
3. Eponychium
4. Body of nail
5. Hyponychium

Figure 9.4 Types of skin glands.

1. Hair
2. Sebaceous gland
3. Epidermis
4. Dermis
5. Hypodermis
6. Hair follicle
7. Apocrine sweat gland
8. Eccrine sweat gland

Exercise 10 Structure of Bone Tissue

INTRODUCTION

This exercise is designed to introduce students to the structure of bone tissue. Students are also introduced to the surface features of bone and relevant terminology. A knowledge of these features can help students understand how bones articulate with each other, as well as how muscles attach to bone.

MATERIALS

1. Histological slides of bone
2. Longitudinally sectioned femur showing compact and spongy bone
3. Colored pencils
4. Reference text

KEY TO LABELING AND TABLE EXERCISES

Figure 10.1 A section through the skull showing diploe.

1. Suture
2. Spongy bone
3. Inner compact bone
4. Outer compact bone

Figure 10.2 A diagram of a long bone shown in longitudinal section.

1. Proximal epiphysis
2. Spongy bone
3. Compact bone
4. Medullary cavity
5. Endosteum
6. Periosteum
7. Nutrient foramen
8. Nutrient vessel
9. Epiphyseal plate
10. Distal epiphysis
11. Diaphysis

Figure 10.3 The histological structure of bone tissue: (*a*) a section cut out of the femur; (*b*) an enlarged section of bone showing compact and spongy bone tissue; (*c*) an osteon (haversian system).

1. Periosteum
2. Osteon
3. Osteocyte
4. Lamellae (matrix)
5. Lacuna
6. Canaliculi
7. Central canal
8. Spongy bone
9. Compact bone

Table 10.1 Surface features of bones

Large, rounded articulating knob
Prominent, rounded articulating end of bone
Flattened or shallow articulating surface
Small, rounded process
Large roughened process
Massive process found only on the femur
Sharp, slender process
Narrow, ridgelike projection
Projection above condyle

Flattened or shallow basin
Narrow slitlike opening
Tubelike passageway into bone
Rounded opening through bone
Cavity or hollow space in bone

Exercise 11 Skeletal System: The Axial Skeleton

INTRODUCTION

This exercise is designed to introduce students to the bones and surface features of the axial skeleton. Students will find learning the skeleton much easier when looking at actual bones, and so laboratory time can be a valuable experience. The protective role of the axial skeleton should be emphasized during the exercise.

MATERIALS

1. Articulated and disarticulated skeletons
2. Skull of a fetus showing fontanels
3. Colored pencils
4. Reference text

KEY TO LABELING EXERCISES

Figure 11.1 The fetal skull.

1. Anterior fontanel
2. Sagittal suture
3. Posterior fontanel
4. Lambdoidal suture
5. Posterolateral fontanel
6. Squamosal suture
7. Anterolateral fontanel
8. Coronal suture

Figure 11.2 A lateral view of the skull.

1. Parietal bone
2. Lambdoidal suture
3. Squamosal suture
4. Temporal bone
5. Occipital bone
6. Superior nuchal line
7. External acoustic meatus
8. Mastoid part of temporal bone
9. Styloid process of temporal bone
10. Mandibular fossa
11. Zygomatic process of temporal bone
12. Coronal suture
13. Frontal bone
14. Sphenoid bone
15. Zygomatic bone

Figure 11.3 An inferior aspect of the skull (with the lower jaw removed).

1. Premolar teeth
2. Molar teeth
3. Zygomatic bone
4. Zygomatic arch
5. Vomer
6. Mandibular fossa
7. Styloid process of temporal bone
8. Occipital condyle
9. Mastoid part of temporal bone
10. Mastoid foramen
11. Occipital bone
12. External occipital protuberance
13. Incisor teeth
14. Canine tooth
15. Incisive fossa
16. Palatine process of maxilla
17. Palatine bone
18. Greater palatine foramen
19. Pterygoid process of sphenoid bone
20. Foramen lacerum
21. Foramen ovale
22. Carotid canal
23. Jugular foramen
24. Stylomastoid foramen
25. Foramen magnum
26. Superior nuchal line

Figure 11.4 The floor of the cranial cavity.

1. Cribriform plate of ethmoid bone
2. Sphenoid bone
3. Optic foramen
4. Foramen rotundum
5. Foramen spinosum
6. Internal acoustic meatus
7. Foramen magnum
8. Crista galli of ethmoid bone
9. Greater wing of sphenoid bone
10. Sella turcica
11. Foramen ovale
12. Jugular foramen

Figure 11.5 Radiographs of the skull showing paranasal sinuses: (*a*) an anteroposterior view; (*b*) a right lateral view.

a.
1. Ethmoidal sinus
2. Frontal sinus
3. Sphenoidal sinus
4. Maxillary sinus

b.
1. Frontal sinus
2. Sphenoidal sinus
3. Ethmoidal sinus
4. Maxillary sinus

Figure 11.6 An anterior view of the skull.

1. Frontal bone
2. Parietal bone
3. Coronal suture
4. Supraorbital foramen
5. Supraorbital margin
6. Sphenoid bone
7. Ethmoid bone
8. Maxilla
9. Infraorbital foramen
10. Perpendicular plate of ethmoid bone
11. Maxilla
12. Premolar teeth
13. Mandible
14. Mental foramen
15. Temporal bone
16. Zygomatic process of frontal bone
17. Superior orbital fissure
18. Nasal bone
19. Lacrimal bone
20. Zygomatic bone
21. Nasal concha
22. Vomer
23. Ramus of mandible
24. Mandible
25. Angle of mandible
26. Molar teeth
27. Canine tooth
28. Incisor teeth

Figure 11.7 The mandible.

1. Coronoid process
2. Mandibular foramen
3. Alveolar margin
4. Mental foramen
5. Body of mandible
6. Condyloid process
7. Mandibular notch
8. Ramus of mandible
9. Angle of mandible

Figure 11.8 Views of the hyoid bone: (*a*) anterior; (*b*) its position in the anterior neck region.

1. Greater cornu
2. Lesser cornu
3. Body
4. Hyoid bone

Figure 11.9 The three auditory ossicles within the middle ear cavity.

1. Malleus
2. Incus
3. Stapes

Figure 11.10 The vertebral column of an adult, showing curvatures and regions.

1. Intervertebral discs
2. Intervertebral foramina
3. Sacrum
4. Coccyx
5. Cervical curvature
6. Thoracic curvature
7. Lumbar curvature
8. Pelvic curvature

Figure 11.11 Cervical vertebrae: (*a*) a typical cervical vertebra; (*b*) the atlas and axis as they articulate.

a.
1. Bifid spinous process
2. Superior articular process
3. Vertebral foramen
4. Lamina
5. Pedicle
6. Transverse foramen
7. Body

b.
1. Anterior arch of atlas
2. Superior articular surface for occipital condyles
3. Transverse foramina
4. Spinous process of axis
5. Transverse processes
6. Dens (odontoid process)

Figure 11.12 Thoracic vertebrae: (*a*) a right lateral view; (b) a superior view.

1. Fovea
2. Fovea
3. Fovea
4. Pedicle
5. Fovea for tubercle of rib
6. Transverse process
7. Inferior articular process
8. Fovea
9. Body
10. Intervertebral disc
11. Spinous process
12. Fovea
13. Vertebral foramen
14. Superior articular process
15. Body
16. Pedicle
17. Lamina

Figure 11.13 Lumbar vertebrae: (*a*) a superior view; (*b*) a right lateral view.

a.
1. Vertebral foramen
2. Superior articular process
3. Spinous process
4. Body
5. Pedicle
6. Transverse process
7. Lamina

b.
1. Superior articular process
2. Transverse process
3. Spinous process
4. Inferior articular process
5. Intervertebral disc
6. Body

Figure 11.14 The sacrum and coccyx: (*a*) an anterior view; (*b*) a posterior view.

1. Superior articular process
2. Sacral promontory
3. Transverse lines
4. Pelvic foramen
5. Transverse process
6. Coccyx
7. Superior portion of sacral canal
8. Sacral tuberosity
9. Auricular surface
10. Median sacral crest
11. Coccyx
12. Inferior portion of sacral canal
13. Posterior sacral foramina

Figure 11.15 The rib cage.

1. Jugular notch
2. Costal cartilage
3. Costal notches
4. True ribs
5. False ribs
6. Floating ribs
7. Clavicular notch
8. Manubrium
9. Body
10. Xiphoid process
11. Intercostal spaces
12. Sternum

Figure 11.16 The structure of a rib.

1. Articular facets
2. Head
3. Neck
4. Articular facet
5. Tubercle
6. Angle
7. Costal groove
8. Shaft
9. Costal cartilage

INTRODUCTION

This exercise is designed to introduce students to the bones of the appendicular skeleton. Particular attention should be paid to diagnostic features on the bones. Students will find this important when they learn the origins and insertions of muscles. A comparison of the functional adaptations of the bones of the upper and lower extremities would also be appropriate at this time.

MATERIALS

1. Articulated and disarticulated skeletons
2. Male pelvis and female pelvis
3. Chart of the skeletal system
4. Radiographic viewing box with assorted radiographs
5. Colored pencils
6. Reference text

KEY TO LABELING EXERCISES

Figure 12.1 The right clavicle: (*a*) a superior view; (*b*) an inferior view.

1. Conoid tubercle
2. Acromial extremity
3. Acromial extremity
4. Sternal extremity
5. Sternal extremity
6. Costal tuberosity
7. Conoid tubercle

Figure 12.2 The right scapula: (*a*) an anterior view; (*b*) a posterior view.

1. Coracoid process
2. Acromion
3. Glenoid cavity
4. Subscapular fossa
5. Lateral border
6. Superior angle
7. Inferior angle
8. Acromion
9. Coracoid
10. Scapular notch
11. Superior border
12. Superior angle
13. Supraspinous fossa
14. Spine
15. Medial border
16. Infraspinous fossa
17. Inferior angle

Figure 12.3 The right humerus: (*a*) an anterior view; (*b*) a posterior view.

1. Lesser tubercle
2. Greater tubercle
3. Intertubercular groove
4. Head
5. Anatomical neck
6. Surgical neck
7. Nutrient foramen
8. Deltoid tuberosity
9. Coronoid fossa
10. Lateral epicondyle
11. Capitulum
12. Olecranon fossa
13. Medial epicondyle
14. Trochlea

Figure 12.4 Right radius and ulna (anterior view). A cross section showing the binding interosseous ligament is also shown.

1. Head of radius
2. Neck of radius
3. Radial tuberosity
4. Shaft of radius
5. Styloid process of radius
6. Olecranon
7. Trochlear notch
8. Coronoid process
9. Shaft of ulna
10. Interosseous crest
11. Interosseous ligament
12. Head of ulna
13. Styloid process of ulna

Figure 12.5 The right radius and ulna (a posterior view).

1. Olecranon
2. Shaft of ulna
3. Styloid process of ulna
4. Trochlear notch
5. Coronoid process
6. Head of radius
7. Neck of radius
8. Radial tuberosity
9. Shaft of radius
10. Styloid process of radius

Figure 12.6 The bones of the right hand (a posterior view).

1. Trapezoid
2. Trapezium
3. Scaphoid
4. Lunate
5. Distal row
6. Middle row
7. Proximal row
8. Capitate
9. Hamate
10. Triquetrum
11. Pisiform

Figure 12.7 The bones of the right hand (an anterior view).

1. Middle row
2. Head of metacarpal bone
3. Shaft of metacarpal bone
4. Base of metacarpal bone
5. Hamate
6. Triquetrum
7. Pisiform
8. Capitate
9. Lunate
10. Distal row
11. Proximal row
12. Trapezoid
13. Trapezium
14. Scaphoid

Figure 12.8 An anterior view of the pelvic girdle.

1. Iliac fossa
2. Anterior superior iliac spine
3. Anterior inferior iliac spine
4. Acetabular notch
5. Body of ischium
6. Symphysis pubis
7. Pubic tubercle
8. Obturator foramen
9. Spine of ischium
10. Acetabulum
11. Sacroiliac joint
12. Ilium
13. Iliac crest

Figure 12.9 The lateral aspect of the right os coxa.

1. Iliac crest
2. Ilium
3. Posterior superior iliac spine
4. Posterior inferior iliac spine
5. Greater sciatic notch
6. Acetabulum
7. Spine of ischium
8. Lesser sciatic notch
9. Ischium
10. Ischial tuberosity
11. Anterior superior iliac spine
12. Anterior inferior iliac spine
13. Superior ramus of pubis
14. Body of pubis
15. Inferior ramus of pubis
16. Obturator foramen
17. Ramus of ischium

Figure 12.10 The right femur: (*a*) an anterior view; (*b*) a posterior view.

1. Intertrochanteric line
2. Lateral epicondyle
3. Patellar surface
4. Head
5. Neck
6. Lesser trochanter
7. Shaft
8. Medial epicondyle
9. Greater trochanter
10. Intertrochanteric crest
11. Linea aspera
12. Intercondylar fossa
13. Condyles

Figure 12.11 The right tibia and patella: (*a*) an anterior view; (*b*) a posterior view.

1. Base of patella
2. Apex of patella
3. Intercondylar eminence
4. Tibial tuberosity
5. Anterior crest
6. Medial malleolus
7. Articular facets
8. Condyles
9. Head of fibula
10. Lateral malleolus

Figure 12.12 The right foot: (*a*) a superior view; (*b*) an inferior view.

1. Distal row
2. Head
3. Body
4. Base
5. Medial cuneiform
6. Intermediate cuneiform
7. Lateral cuneiform
8. Scaphoid
9. Talus
10. Middle row
11. Proximal row
12. Cuboid bone
13. Calcaneus
14. Tuberosity of calcaneus

Exercise 13 Articulations

INTRODUCTION

This exercise is designed to introduce students to articulations. The three types of joints as well as the structure of a synovial joint are discussed. Students are also introduced to the types of movements possible at synovial joints. The dissection of a beef or pig knee joint can be very effective to introduce students to joint structures. A discussion of the different types of levers found in the body could be helpful to the students in understanding how joints and the muscles spanning these joints function together to cause movements.

MATERIALS

1. Articulated skeleton
2. Disarticulated skeleton
3. Skull of an infant and of an adult
4. Radiographic viewing box with assorted radiographs
5. Colored pencils
6. Reference text
7. Fresh beef or pig knee joint and dissection instruments

KEY TO LABELING EXERCISES

Figure 13.1 Various joints of the body.

1. Suture
2. Symphyses
3. Symphyses
4. Syndesmosis
5. Condyloid joint
6. Gliding joint
7. Pivot joint
8. Pivot joint
9. Saddle joint
10. Ball-and-socket

Figure 13.2 A synovial joint is represented by this diagrammatic lateral view of the knee joint.

1. Articular cartilage
2. Meniscus
3. Joint capsule
4. Synovial membrane
5. Prepatellar bursa
6. Infrapatellar bursa

Figure 13.3 Movements at synovial joints.

1. Hyperextension
2. Extension
3. Flexion
4. Rotation
5. Adduction
6. Pronation
7. Supination
8. Dorsiflexion
9. Plantar flexion
10. Abduction
11. Eversion
12. Inversion
13. Circumduction
14. Protraction
15. Retraction

Exercise 14 Neural Control of Skeletal Muscle Contraction

INTRODUCTION

This exercise is designed to introduce students to skeletal muscle contraction. In this exercise, students will pithed a frog, prepare recording equipment, and then stimulate the sciatic nerve. By changing the stimulus voltage, students will be able to see a threshold stimulus cause muscle contraction. Exercises using animals are very effective for teaching physiological principles, since students can see the principle in action. However, it is important to treat the laboratory animal considerately. Caution the students not to overstimulate the frog muscle early in the lab, since there is no way to replenish the energy stores in the muscle.

MATERIALS
1. Frogs
2. Surgical scissors, forceps, sharp probes and pins, dissecting trays, glass probes
3. Recording equipment (either a kymograph or an electrical recorder, such as a Physiograph), electrical stimulators
4. Straight pins bent into Z shapes, thread
5. Myograph transducer (if Physiograph is used)
6. Frog Ringer's solution; dissolve 6 g NaCl, 0.075 g KCl, 0.10 g $CaCl_2$, and 0.10 g $NaHCO_3$ in 1 liter of water

Exercise 15 Summation, Tetanus, and Fatigue

INTRODUCTION
This exercise is designed to introduce students to principles of skeletal muscle contraction such as summation, tetanus, and fatigue. In this exercise, a frog gastrocnemius muscle is stimulated with increased voltage to demonstrate summation, with increased frequency to demonstrate tetanus, and then continually to cause fatigue. This procedure can then be repeated on a human subject. This exercise can be combined with exercise 14, since both experiments use the same setup with the frogs.

MATERIALS
1. Frogs
2. Equipment and setup used in exercise 14
3. Electrocardiograph plates and electrolyte gel
4. Alternative equipment: Physiogrip™(Intelitool, Inc.) with IBM or Apple computer and squarewave stimulator

Exercise 16 Muscles of the Head and Neck

INTRODUCTION
This exercise is designed to introduce students to the muscles of the head and neck. Remind your students that many of the muscles to be learned can be palpated and contracted. Learning the origin and insertion of each muscle will also help the student to understand its action, as well as its name.

MATERIALS
1. Drawing pencils
2. Laboratory manikin
3. Wall charts of human muscles
4. Articulated human skeleton
5. Reference text and atlas
6. Colored pencils

KEY TO LABELING AND TABLE EXERCISES
Figure 16.1 Superficial facial muscles.
1. Temporalis
2. Occipitalis
3. Frontalis
4. Orbicularis oculi
5. Corrugator
6. Nasalis
7. Levator labii superioris
8. Orbicularis oris
9. Zygomaticus
10. Buccinator
11. Depressor labii inferioris
12. Mentalis
13. Depressor anguli oris
14. Risorius
15. Platysma
16. Masseter

Figure 16.2 Muscles of mastication: (*a*) a superficial view; (*b*) a deep view.

1. Temporalis
2. Masseter
3. Lateral pterygoid
4. Medial pterygoid

Figure 16.3 Muscles of the neck.

1. Trapezius
2. Stylohyoid
3. Posterior belly of digastric
4. Hyoglossus
5. Mylohyoid
6. Anterior belly of digastric
7. Thyrohyoid
8. Omohyoid
9. Sternohyoid
10. Middle pharyngeal constrictor
11. Sternocleidomastoid

Table 16.1 Muscles of facial expression

Compresses cheek
Draws eyebrows toward midline
Depresses lower lip
Wrinkles forehead and moves scalp
Elevates upper lip
Elevates and protrudes lower lip
Compresses nostrils
Moves scalp backwards
Closes eye
Closes and purses lips
Depresses lower lip
Draws angle of mouth laterally
Depresses corner of mouth
Elevates corner of mouth

Table 16.2 Muscles of mastication

Elevates mandible
Elevates mandible
Elevates mandible and moves mandible laterally
Protracts mandible

Table 16.3 Muscles of the neck

Turns head to side; flexes neck and head
Elevates scapula, draws head back, adducts scapula, braces shoulder
Opens mouth; elevates hyoid
Depresses side of tongue
Elevates hyoid bone and floor of mouth
Elevates and retracts tongue
Depresses hyoid
Depresses hyoid
Depresses hyoid; elevates thyroid

Exercise 17 Muscles of the Pectoral Girdle and Upper Extremity

INTRODUCTION

This exercise is designed to introduce students to the muscles of the pectoral girdle and upper extremity. Remind your students that many of the muscles to be learned can be palpated and contracted. Learning the origin and insertion of each muscle will also help the student to understand its action, as well as its name.

MATERIALS

1. Drawing pencils
2. Laboratory manikin
3. Wall charts of human muscles
4. Articulated human skeleton
5. Reference text and atlas
6. Colored pencils

KEY TO LABELING AND TABLE EXERCISES

Figure 17.1 Anterior muscles of the neck and thorax (superficial muscles removed from the right side).

1. Pectoralis major
2. Latissimus dorsi
3. Serratus anterior
4. Deltoid
5. Biceps brachii

Figure 17.2 Posterior muscles of the trunk (dorsal aspect; superficial muscles removed from the right side).

1. Trapezius
2. Deltoid
3. Infraspinatus
4. Teres minor
5. Teres major
6. Latissimus dorsi
7. Levator scapula
8. Supraspinatus
9. Rhomboideus minor
10. Teres major
11. Rhomboideus major

Figure 17.3 Deep muscles of the thorax and brachium.

1. Subclavius
2. Coracobrachialis
3. Subscapularis
4. Long head of biceps brachii
5. Teres major
6. Latissimus dorsi
7. Short head of biceps brachii
8. Brachialis
9. Serratus anterior
10. Pectoralis minor

Figure 17.4 Right shoulder and brachium: (*a*) an anterior view; (*b*) a posterior view.

1. Long head of biceps brachii
2. Short head of biceps brachii
3. Brachialis
4. Brachioradialis
5. Long head of triceps brachii
6. Medial head of triceps brachii
7. Lateral head of triceps brachii

Figure 17.6 Deep muscles of the forearm: (*a*) rotators; (*b*) flexors; (*c*) extensors.

1. Pronator teres
2. Flexor carpi radialis
3. Superficial digital flexor
4. Flexor pollicis longus
5. Palmaris longus (cut)
6. Flexor carpi ulnaris
7. Extensor carpi ulnaris
8. Abductor pollicis longus
9. Extensor pollicis longus
10. Extensor carpi radialis longus
11. Extensor digitorum

Table 17.1 Muscles that act on the pectoral girdle

Pulls scapula forward and downward
Pulls scapula forward and downward
Elevates scapula, draws head back, adducts scapula, braces shoulder
Elevates scapula
Elevates and adducts scapula
Elevates and adducts scapula
Draws clavicle downward

Table 17.2 Muscles that move the humerus

Extends, adducts, and rotates humerus medially; retracts shoulder
Flexes, adducts, and rotates arm medially
Flexes and adducts shoulder joint
Abducts arm; extends or flexes humerus
Rotates arm laterally
Rotates arm medially
Abducts and laterally rotates humerus
Extends humerus, or adducts and rotates arm medially
Rotates arm laterally

Table 17.3 Muscles that act on the forearm

Flexes and supinates forearm and hand
Flexes forearm
Flexes forearm
Extends forearm

Table 17.4 Muscles that move the wrist, hand, and fingers

Pronates forearm
Flexes and abducts hand
Flexes and adducts wrist
Flexes wrist, hand, and digits
Flexes thumb
Flexes wrist
Abducts thumb and hand
Extends and abducts hand
Extends and abducts hand
Extends and adducts wrist
Extends wrist and digits
Extends thumb; abducts hand

INTRODUCTION

This exercise is designed to introduce students to the muscles of the trunk and lower extremity. Remind your students that many of the muscles to be learned can be palpated and contracted. Learning the origin and insertion of each muscle will also help the student to understand its action, as well as its name.

MATERIALS

1. Drawing pencils
2. Laboratory manikin
3. Wall charts of human muscles
4. Articulated human skeleton
5. Reference text and atlas
6. Colored pencils

KEY TO LABELING AND TABLE EXERCISES

Figure 18.1 Muscles of the anterior abdominal wall.

1. Internal abdominal oblique
2. Transverse abdominis
3. Sheath of rectus abdominis
4. Linea alba
5. External abdominal oblique
6. Rectus abdominis

Figure 18.2 Muscles of the vertebral column.

1. Splenius capitis
2. Spinalis thoracis
3. Quadratus lumborum
4. Semispinalis capitis
5. Longissimus thoracis
6. Iliocostalis thoracis
7. External abdominal oblique

Figure 18.3 Anterior pelvic muscles.

1. Costal portion of diaphragm
2. Spinal portion of diaphragm
3. Quadratus lumborum
4. Inguinal ligament
5. Psoas major
6. Illacus

Figure 18.5 The deep gluteal muscles (a posterior view).

1. Gluteus maximus
2. Semimembranosus
3. Semitendinosus
4. Gluteus medius
5. Gluteus minimus
6. Long head of biceps femoris

Figure 18.6 Muscles of the thigh (an anterior view).

1. Tensor fasciae latae
2. Sartorius
3. Rectus femoris
4. Vastus lateralis
5. Pectineus
6. Adductor longus
7. Adductor magnus
8. Vastus medialis

Figure 18.7 Muscles of the thigh (a posterior view).

1. Adductor magnus
2. Gracilis
3. Semitendinosus
4. Semimembranosus
5. Sartorius
6. Long head of biceps femoris

Figure 18.9 Anterior crural muscles.

1. Peroneus longus
2. Tibialis anterior
3. Extensor digitorum longus
4. Peroneus brevis
5. Extensor hallucis longus
6. Gastrocnemius
7. Soleus
8. Tibia
9. Flexor digitorum longus

Figure 18.10 Lateral crural muscles.

1. Gastrocnemius
2. Soleus
3. Peroneus longus
4. Tibialis anterior
5. Extensor digitorum longus
6. Peroneus brevis
7. Peroneus tertius

Figure 18.11 Posterior crural muscles and the popliteal fossa.

1. Medial head of gastrocnemius
2. Plantaris
3. Lateral head of gastrocnemius
4. Soleus
5. Tendo calcaneus

Table 18.1 Muscles of the abdominal wall

Compresses abdomen; lateral rotation
Compresses abdomen; lateral rotation
Compresses abdomen
Flexes vertebral column

Table 18.2 Anterior and posterior muscles that move the thigh at the hip

Flexes and rotates thigh laterally; flexes vertebral column
Flexes and rotates thigh laterally; flexes vertebral column
Extends and rotates thigh laterally
Abducts and rotates thigh medially
Abducts and rotates thigh medially
Abducts thigh

Table 18.3 Anterior thigh muscles that move the leg

Flexes leg and thigh, abducts thigh, rotates thigh laterally, and rotates leg medially
Extends leg at knee
Extends leg at knee
Extends leg at knee
Extends leg at knee
Extends leg at knee

Table 18.4 Medial thigh muscles that move the leg

Adducts thigh; flexes and rotates leg at knee
Adducts and flexes thigh
Adducts, flexes, and laterally rotates thigh
Adducts, flexes, and laterally rotates thigh
Adducts, flexes, and laterally rotates thigh

Table 18.5 Posterior thigh muscles that move the leg

Flexes leg at knee; extends and laterally rotates thigh at hip
Flexes leg at knee; extends and medially rotates thigh at hip
Flexes leg at knee; extends and medially rotates thigh at hip

Table 18.6 Muscles of the leg that move the ankle, foot, and toes

Dorsiflexion of ankle and inversion of foot
Extends digits II-V and dorsiflexes foot
Extends hallux and assists dorsiflexion of foot
Dorsiflexes and everts foot
Plantar flexes and everts foot
Plantar flexes and everts foot
Plantar flexes foot; flexes knee

Plantar flexes foot
Plantar flexes foot
Flexes distal phalanx of hallux
Flexes distal phalanx of digits II-V
Plantar flexes and inverts foot; supports arches

Exercise 19 Cat Musculature

INTRODUCTION

This exercise is designed for laboratories that do not have human cadavers. The best way to learn anatomy is to dissect a laboratory specimen. Human cadavers are ideal for human anatomy courses but are not always available, nor are they practical for all courses. Often embalmed cats are dissected instead. Despite the definite anatomical differences between cats and humans, there are far greater similarities than differences; the dissection of cats is thus a suitable substitute for human cadaver dissections.

MATERIALS

1. Embalmed cats
2. Dissecting trays
3. Dissecting instruments
4. Plastic bags and name tags
5. Muslin cloth
6. Reference text

Exercise 20 Brain and Cranial Nerves

INTRODUCTION

This exercise is designed to introduce students to the structure of the brain and the cranial nerves. Examination of laboratory specimens and models can help the students develop a working knowledge of neuroanatomy. The instructions for the removal of the brain from a sheep or cat head are also presented and provide a means for students to learn more about the anatomy of the brain. Students should be cautious in using the bone saw during this exercise. Extra care should also be taken in removing the brain from the skull in order to preserve as many of the cranial nerves as possible.

MATERIALS

1. Dissecting instruments and trays
2. Preserved mammalian brains (human, if available; otherwise, sheep or cat)
3. Colored pencils
4. (Optional) Preserved cat or fresh sheep head, autopsy saw, large screwdriver

KEY TO LABELING EXERCISES

Figure 20.1 The developmental sequence of the brain: (*a*) undifferentiated; (*b*) the three-region brain; (*c*) the five-region brain.

1. Neural tube
2. Prosencephalon
3. Diencephalon
4. Telencephalon
5. Mesencephalon
6. Rhombencephalon
7. Mesencephalon
8. Metencephalon
9. Myelencephalon

Figure 20.2 The cranial meninges and the layers of the cerebrum as shown in a coronal section through the cranium and brain.

1. Scalp
2. Periosteum
3. Bone
4. Dura mater
5. Arachnoid mater
6. Pia mater
7. Subarachnoid space
8. Falx cerebri

Figure 20.3 The cerebrum and cerebellum: (*a*) a lateral view; (*b*) a superior view.

1. Parietal lobe
2. Parietooccipital fissure
3. Occipital lobe
4. Cerebellar hemisphere
5. Central sulcus
6. Sulcus
7. Convolutions
8. Gyrus
9. Frontal lobe
10. Lateral fissure
11. Temporal lobe
12. Longitudinal fissure
13. Left hemisphere
14. Vermis
15. Right hemisphere

Figure 20.4 An inferior view of the brain and cranial nerves.

1. Olfactory bulb
2. Longitudinal fissure
3. Olfactory tract
4. Optic chiasma
5. Oculomotor nerve
6. Mammillary body
7. Trochlear nerve
8. Trigeminal nerve
9. Abducens nerve
10. Facial nerve
11. Medulla oblongata
12. Hypoglossal nerve
13. Cerebellum
14. Optic nerve
15. Ophthalmic branch of the trigeminal nerve
16. Maxillary branch of the trigeminal nerve
17. Mandibular branch of the trigeminal nerve
18. Pons
19. Vestibulocochlear nerve
20. Glossopharyngeal nerve
21. Vagus nerve
22. Accessory nerve

Figure 20.5 An inferior view of the arteries that supply blood to the brain.

1. Internal carotid a.
2. Middle cerebral a.
3. Cerebral arterial circle
4. Superior cerebellar a.
5. Basilar a.
6. Vertebral a.
7. Anterior cerebral a.
8. Posterior cerebral a.

Figure 20.6 A midsagittal section of the brain.

1. Corpus callosum
2. Septum pellucidum
3. Cerebrum
4. Genu of corpus callosum
5. Thalamus
6. Optic chiasma
7. Infundibulum
8. Pituitary gland
9. Hypothalamus
10. Mammillary body
11. Pons
12. Medulla oblongata
13. Splenium of corpus callosum
14. Pineal body
15. Corpora quadrigemina
16. Arbor vitae
17. Cerebellum

Figure 20.7 A midsagittal section of the brain showing the ventricles of the brain and the direction of flow of the cerebrospinal fluid.

1. Lateral ventricle
2. Interventricular foramen
3. Third ventricle
4. Mesenchephalic aqueduct
5. Fourth ventricle
6. Choroid plexus of third ventricle
7. Arachnoid villi
8. Subarachnoid space

Exercise 21 Spinal Cord, Spinal Nerves, and Spinal Reflexes

INTRODUCTION

This exercise is designed to introduce students to the structure of the spinal cord and to spinal reflexes. This exercise demonstrates tests for spinal nerve stretch reflexes and referred pain. Observing histological slides of nervous tissue will help students understand the structures of the spinal cord and spinal nerves.

MATERIALS

1. Microscope
2. Histological slides of a spinal cord and spinal nerve
3. Rubber mallets
4. Reference text
5. Optional: Flexicomp™(Intelitool, Inc.) with IBM or Apple computer

KEY TO LABELING EXERCISES

Figure 21.1 The spinal cord and plexuses.

1. Cervical plexus
2. Brachial plexus
3. Radial nerve
4. Median nerve
5. Ulnar nerve
6. Dura mater
7. Cauda equina
8. Lumbosacral plexus
9. Sciatic nerve

Figure 21.2 A cross section of the spinal cord.

1. Posterior median sulcus
2. Posterior horn
3. Lateral horn
4. Anterior horn
5. Central canal
6. Anterior median fissure
7. Gray matter
8. Anterior root
9. White matter
10. Posterior root
11. Posterior root ganglion

Figure 21.3 The knee-jerk reflex, an example of a monosynaptic stretch reflex.

1. Cell body of sensory neuron
2. Sensory neuron
3. Alpha motor neuron
4. Skeletal muscle fibers
5. Spindle apparatus

Exercise 22 Cutaneous Receptors

INTRODUCTION

This exercise is designed to introduce students to the types of cutaneous receptors found throughout the body. By mapping temperature and touch receptors, as well as sensory adaptation, students will have a better understanding of how receptors function. This exercise could be combined with exercises 23, 24, and 25 for an entire laboratory period devoted to the sensory systems of the body.

MATERIALS

1. Thin bristles
2. Cold and warm metal rods
3. Calipers
4. Cold and warm water baths
5. Colored pencils

KEY TO LABELING EXERCISES

Figure 22.1 Diagrammatic section of skin showing cutaneous receptors.

1. Organ of Ruffini
2. Root hair plexus
3. Lamellated pacinian corpuscle
4. Free nerve endings
5. Corpuscle of touch
6. Bulb of Kraus

Exercise 23 Eyes and Vision

INTRODUCTION

This exercise is designed to introduce students to the anatomy of the eye, and to the processes involved in vision. Students may also find dissection of a beef or sheep eye useful in learning the structures of the eye. This exercise could be combined with exercises 22, 24, and 25 for an entire laboratory period devoted to the sensory systems of the body.

MATERIALS

1. Fresh or preserved beef or sheep eyes
2. Dissecting instruments and trays
3. Snellen eye chart and astigmatism chart
4. Wire screen and meter stick
5. Opthalmoscope

KEY TO LABELING EXERCISES

Figure 23.1 Ocular muscles of the left eyeball: (*a*) a lateral view; (*b*) a superior view.

a.
1. Trochlea
2. Superior oblique muscle
3. Levator palpebrae
4. Superior rectus muscle
5. Medial rectus muscle
6. Lateral rectus muscle
7. Inferior rectus muscle
8. Inferior oblique muscle

b.
1. Trochlea
2. Superior oblique muscle
3. Levator palpebrae

Figure 23.2 The internal anatomy of the eyeball.

1. Superior rectus muscle
2. Sclera
3. Choroid layer
4. Retina
5. Optic disc
6. Optic nerve
7. Inferior rectus muscle
8. Conjunctiva
9. Ciliary body
10. Posterior chamber
11. Cornea
12. Anterior chamber
13. Pupil
14. Lens
15. Iris
16. Posterior chamber
17. Suspensory ligament
18. Vitreous chamber

Exercise 24 Ears and Hearing

INTRODUCTION

This exercise is designed to introduce students to the anatomy of the ear and the processes involved in hearing. Studying the structure of the ear from models, as well as from sections of the petrous portion of the temporal bone, could be helpful to students. This exercise could be combined with exercises 22, 23, and 25 for an entire laboratory period devoted to the sensory systems of the body.

MATERIALS

1. Tuning forks
2. Rubber mallets
3. Reference text
4. Colored pencils

KEY TO LABELING EXERCISES

Figure 24.1 The ear.

1. Auricle
2. Malleus
3. Semicircular canals
4. Incus
5. Stapes
6. Vestibular nerve
7. Cochlear nerve
8. Round window
9. Cochlea
10. Tympanic cavity
11. Auditory canal
12. Vestibule
13. Tympanic membrane
14. External auditory canal

Figure 24.2 Structures of the inner ear (*a*); the spiral organ (organ of Corti) (*b*).

1. Hair cell of semicircular canal
2. Semicircular canal
3. Vestibule
4. Membranous labyrinth
5. Bony labyrinth
6. Vestibular ducts
7. Cochlea
8. Scala vestibuli
9. Cochlear duct
10. Scala tympani
11. Vestibular membrane
12. Tectorial membrane
13. Hair cells
14. Cochlear nerve
15. Basilar membrane
16. Spiral organ (organ of Corti)

Exercise 25 Taste

INTRODUCTION

This exercise is designed to introduce students to the structure of the tongue and tongue papillae and how they function in taste. This exercise could be combined with exercises 22, 23, and 24 for an entire laboratory period devoted to the sensory systems of the body.

MATERIALS

1. Cotton-tipped applicator sticks
2. Solutions of 5% sucrose, 1% acetic acid, 5% sodium chloride, and 0.5% quinine sulfate

KEY TO LABELING EXERCISES

Figure 25.1 Papillae of the tongue and associated taste buds.

1. Papillae
2. Taste buds
3. Sensory fiber
4. Gustatory cell
5. Supportive cell
6. Taste pore
7. Gustatory hair

Exercise 26 Endocrine System

INTRODUCTION

This exercise is designed to introduce students to the glands of the endocrine system and the hormones produced by each gland. The endocrine system works closely with the nervous system to maintain homeostasis and therefore is very important in the physiology of body systems. Students will benefit from examining histological slides of each gland. It should also be emphasized that the organs of the endocrine system are not the only organs of the body that secrete hormones.

MATERIALS

1. Microscopes
2. Prepared histological slides
3. Human torso model, human brain model, skull
4. Reference text and atlases
5. Colored pencils

KEY TO LABELING EXERCISES

Figure 26.1 The pituitary gland.

1. Infundibulum
2. Pars nervosa
3. Adenohypophysis (anterior lobe)
4. Pars intermediate lobe

Figure 26.2 The thyroid gland.

1. Isthmus
2. Thyroid gland
3. Colloid
4. Thyroid follicle
5. Simple cuboidal epithelial cells

Figure 26.3 A posterior view of the parathyroid glands.

1. Thyroid gland
2. Parathyroid gland

Figure 26.4 The pancreas and the associated pancreatic islets (islets of Langerhans).

1. Tail of pancreas
2. Pancreatic islet (islet of Langerhans)
3. Body of pancreas

Figure 26.5 The structure of the adrenal gland showing the three zones of the adrenal cortex and the adrenal medulla.

1. Adrenal gland
2. Adrenal cortex
3. Adrenal medulla
4. Zona glomerulosa
5. Zona fasciculata
6. Zona reticularis

Figure 26.6 Various endocrine glands.

1. Pineal gland
2. Thymus
3. Placenta
4. Thyroid
5. Ovaries
6. Testes

Figure 26.7 An ovarian follicle with ovum.

1. Corona radiata
2. Granulosa cells
3. Ovum
4. Antrum
5. Ovarian follicle

Figure 26.8 Photomicrograph of a testis.

1. Interstitial (Leydig's) cells
2. Seminiferous tubule
3. Spermatozoa

Exercise 27 Red Blood Cells and Oxygen Transport

INTRODUCTION

This exercise is designed to introduce students to red blood cells. By performing a red blood cell count, measuring a hematocrit, and calculating corpuscular volume and hemoglobin concentration, students will become familiar with red blood cells, their contents, and their functions. Since this exercise deals with blood, be sure to encourage your students to use sterile technique and not to touch anyone's blood but their own. Milking the finger to squeeze out blood will increase the amount of interstitial fluid and cause a lower hematocrit value. Take proper measures to dispose of anything contaminated with blood. This exercise can be combined with exercises 28 and 29 for an entire laboratory period devoted to blood.

MATERIALS
1. Hemocytometer
2. Unopettes (Becton-Dickinson) for manual red blood cell count and hemoglobin measurements
3. Heparinized capillary tubes, clay capillary tube sealant (Seal-ease), microcapillary centrifuge, hematocrit reader
4. Microscope
5. Sterile lancets and 70% alcohol
6. Colorimeter and cuvettes
7. Container for the disposal of blood-containing objects

Exercise 28 Total and Differential White Blood Cell Counts

INTRODUCTION

This exercise is designed to introduce students to white blood cells. By performing total and differential white blood cell counts, students will become familiar with the five types of white blood cells. A discussion of the five types of white blood cells would be helpful at this point. Since this exercise deals with blood, be sure to encourage your students to use sterile technique and not to touch anyone's blood but their own. Take proper measures to dispose of anything contaminated with blood. This exercise can be combined with exercises 27 and 29 for an entire laboratory period devoted to blood.

MATERIALS
1. Microscopes
2. Unopette system for white blood cell counts
3. Lancets, alcohol swabs
4. Wright's stain (or Diff-Quik, Harleco) for differential count
5. Heparinized capillary tubes, glass slides
6. Container for the disposal of blood-containing objects

Exercise 29 Blood Types

INTRODUCTION

This exercise is designed to introduce students to the ABO and Rh blood typing systems. Since blood cells have characteristic antigens on the cell membranes, it is possible to type blood. A discussion of antigens and antibodies may help the students to understand the process of blood typing before they perform their own blood typing. Since this exercise deals with blood, be sure to encourage your students to use sterile technique and not to touch anyone's blood but their own. Take proper measures to dispose of anything contaminated with blood. This exercise can be combined with exercises 27 and 28 for an entire laboratory period devoted to blood.

MATERIALS
1. Glass slides, marking pencils, lancets, and applicator sticks or toothpicks
2. Anti-A, -B, and -Rh sera
3. Slide warmer
4. Container for the disposal of blood-containing objects

Exercise 30 Heart and Arteries

INTRODUCTION

This exercise is designed to introduce students to the structure of the heart and to the principal arteries of the body. The best way to learn the heart and arteries is to examine a dissected laboratory specimen. Human cadavers are best for a human anatomy course, but examining a cat is also very effective. Instructions are given for dissection of a mammalian heart as well as for the dissection of a cat, and students can learn a great deal by performing their own dissections. The names of the principal arteries of the body may be more easily learned if the organs they serve are introduced before learning the artery. For example, if students know that "renal" refers to the kidney, then it is easy for them to learn that the renal artery serves the kidney.

MATERIALS

1. Fresh sheep, pig, or beef heart
2. Dissecting instruments and trays
3. Embalmed cat
4. Heart models and charts of the circulatory system
5. Microscopes
6. Prepared slides of stained heart and blood vessels
7. Reference text

KEY TO LABELING EXERCISES

Figure 30.1 The structure of the heart: (*a*) an anterior view; (*b*) a posterior view; (*c*) an internal view.

a.
1. Superior vena cava
2. Right pulmonary vv.
3. Right atrium
4. Right coronary a.
5. Right ventricle
6. Inferior vena cava
7. Pulmonary trunk
8. Left pulmonary aa.
9. Left pulmonary v.
10. Left atrium
11. Great cardiac v.
12. Anterior interventricular a.
13. Left ~~atrium~~ ventricle

b.
1. Left pulmonary a.
2. Left pulmonary vv.
3. Left atrium
4. Coronary sinus
5. Left ventricle
6. Superior vena cava
7. Right pulmonary a.
8. Right pulmonary vv.
9. Right atrium
10. Inferior vena cava
11. Right ventricle

c.
1. Right pulmonary a.
2. Superior vena cava
3. Right pulmonary v.
4. Pulmonary semilunar valve
5. Right atrium
6. Tricuspid valve
7. Chordae tendineae
8. Inferior vena cava
9. Right ventricle
10. Aortic arch
11. Left pulmonary a.
12. Pulmonary trunk
13. Left pulmonary vv.
14. Left atrium
15. Aortic semilunar valve
16. Bicuspid (mitral) valve
17. Interventricular septum
18. Papillary muscle
19. Left ventricle
20. Descending thoracic aorta

Figure 30.2 The conduction system of the heart.

1. Sinoatrial node (SA node)
2. Atrioventricular node (AV node)
3. Atrioventricular bundle (bundle of His)
4. Conduction myofibers (Purkinje fibers)
5. Right and left bundle branches

Figure 30.8 The structure of (*a*) an artery and (*b*) a vein, showing the relative thickness and composition of the tunicas.

1. Tunica intima
2. Tunica media
3. Tunica externa
4. Valve

Figure 30.9 The principal arteries of the body.

1. External carotid a.
2. Right common carotid a.
3. Right vertebral a.
4. Right subclavian a.
5. Brachiocephalic trunk
6. Axillary a.
7. Ascending aorta
8. Brachial a.
9. Celiac trunk
10. Hepatic a.
11. Superior mesenteric a.
12. Radial a.
13. Ulnar a.
14. External iliac a.
15. Deep femoral a.
16. Femoral a.
17. Popliteal a.
18. Posterior tibial a.
19. Anterior tibial a.
20. Internal carotid a.
21. Left common carotid a.
22. Left subclavian a.
23. Thoracic aorta
24. Left gastric a.
25. Splenic a.
26. Renal aa.
27. Suprarenal a.
28. Gonadal (testicular or ovarian artery)
29. Inferior mesenteric a.
30. Common iliac a.
31. Internal iliac a.

Exercise 31 Veins, Lymphatics, and Fetal Circulation

INTRODUCTION

This exercise is designed to introduce students to veins, lymphatics, and fetal circulation. Just as with exercise 30, students will learn best by examining a dissected specimen. Instructions for observing the venous system of a cat are included in the *Laboratory Manual*. Learning the lymphatic system and fetal circulation off charts and models is very helpful for students. Students should learn veins as structures that return blood to the heart; venules come together to form larger veins.

MATERIALS

1. Colored pencils
2. Embalmed cat, dissecting tray, and dissecting instruments
3. Reference text

KEY TO LABELING EXERCISES

Figure 31.1 Principal veins of the body: the superficial veins are on the left extremities and the deep veins are on the right extremities.

1. Right brachiocephalic v.
2. Superior vena cava
3. Hepatic v.
4. Inferior vena cava
5. Renal v.
6. Testicular (internal spermatic) v. (male)
7. Radial v.
8. Ulnar v.
9. Common iliac v.
10. External iliac v.
11. Internal iliac v.
12. Great saphenous v.
13. Deep femoral v.
14. Femoral v.
15. Popliteal v.
16. Posterior tibial v.
17. Anterior tibial v.
18. External jugular v.
19. Internal jugular v.
20. Subclavian v.
21. Axillary v.
22. Brachial v.
23. Basilic v.
24. Suprarenal v.
25. Cephalic v.
26. Median cubital v.

Figure 31.2 Veins of the thoracic region.

1. External jugular v.
2. Subclavian v.
3. Superior vena cava
4. Axillary v.
5. Brachial v.
6. Basilic v.
7. Azygous v.
8. Internal jugular v.
9. Brachiocephalic v.
10. Cephalic v.
11. Hemiazygos v.
12. Intercostal v.

Figure 31.3 The hepatic portal system.

1. Inferior vena cava
2. Hepatic v.
3. Cystic v.
4. Right gastric v.
5. Hepatic portal vein
6. Right gastroepiploic v.
7. Superior mesenteric v.
8. Left gastric v.
9. Left gastroepiploic v.
10. Splenic v.
11. Pancreatic v.
12. Inferior mesenteric v.

Figure 31.4 Fetal circulation.

1. Foramen ovale
2. Inferior vena cava
3. Umbilical v.
4. Umbilical cord
5. Ductus arteriosus
6. Ductus venosus
7. Umbilical aa.

Figure 31.5 Lymphatic vessels: (*a*) a magnified view of the upper right quadrant showing the lymph drainage of the right breast; (*b*) major lymph drainage of the body.

1. Right lymphatic duct
2. Axillary lymph node
3. Tonsil
4. Thymus
5. Thoracic duct
6. Spleen
7. Cisterna chyli
8. Lumbar lymph node
9. Inguinal lymph node

Exercise 32 Effects of Drugs on the Frog Heart

INTRODUCTION

This exercise is designed to introduce students to the effects of drugs on the heart. Students expose the heart of a frog and then introduce calcium, digitalis, pilocarpine, atropine, potassium, epinephrine, caffeine, and nicotine to the frog heart to see the effects of each drug. Students can determine the effect of the drugs in terms of strength of contraction, rate of contraction, and rate of impulse contraction from the atria to the ventricle.

MATERIALS

1. Frogs, dissecting instruments, and dissecting trays
2. Copper wire and thread
3. Recording apparatus; Physiograph, transducer coupler, and myograph transducer (Narco); or kymograph, kymograph paper, and kerosene burner
4. Ringer's solution (see exercise 14—all drugs should be added to the Ringer's solution, which is used as the solvent); calcium chloride (2.0 g/dl); digitalis (0.2 g/dl); pilocarpine (2.5 g/dl); atropine (2.5 g/dl); potassium chloride (2.0 g/dl); epinephrine (0.01 g/dl); caffeine (saturated; 0.2 g/dl); and nicotine (1.0 g/dl)

Exercise 33 Electrocardiogram

INTRODUCTION

This exercise is designed to introduce students to a method of measuring the electrical activity of the heart — the electrocardiogram. Students will be able to monitor and read ECG recordings after this exercise. This exercise could be combined with exercise 34 for a laboratory period about the electrical activity of the heart.

MATERIALS
1. Electrocardiograph
2. Electrode plates, rubber straps, electrolyte gel or paste
3. Alternative equipment: Cardiocomp™(Intelitool, Inc.), with Apple or IBM (8086 processor) computer

Exercise 34 Mean Electrical Axis of the Ventricles

INTRODUCTION
This exercise is designed to emphasize the use of the ECG to monitor the electrical activity of the heart, particularly the electrical axis of the ventricles. This exercise could be combined with exercise 33 for a laboratory period about the electrical activity of the heart.

MATERIALS
1. Electrocardiograph, or multichannel recorder (e.g., Physiograph) with ECG module; alternatively, a Cardiocomp™(Intelitool, Inc.) may be used with an Apple or IBM computer
2. ECG plates, straps, and gel

Exercise 35 Heart Sounds and Measurement of Blood Pressure

INTRODUCTION
This exercise is designed to introduce students to the sounds produced by the closing of heart valves and to techniques for measuring blood pressure. Remind the students not to pump the cuffs of the sphygmomanometer above 20 mm Hg, because it is very painful for the individual being monitored. It may be effective to explain the mechanics of measuring blood pressure: that the occlusion of the cuff by pressures greater than the systolic pressure prevents the flow of blood through the cuff, but that blood can flow when the systolic pressure is greater than cuff pressure. After this exercise, students should be able to explain and measure blood pressure and monitor heart sounds. It may also be helpful to show students on an ECG where the valves open and close to cause the heart sounds.

MATERIALS
1. Stethoscope
2. Sphygmomanometer

Exercise 36 Cardiovascular System and Physical Fitness

INTRODUCTION
This exercise is designed to introduce students to the effects of exercise on the cardiovascular system. Students will apply techniques learned in exercise 35 to measure blood pressure, and they will learn how to measure pulse rate.

MATERIALS
1. Sphygmomanometer
2. Stethoscope
3. Chair, stair, or platform 18 inches high

Exercise 37 Respiratory System

INTRODUCTION

This exercise is designed to introduce students to the anatomy of the respiratory system. Students must understand the structures of the respiratory system in order to grasp the functions of each structure. The relationship of the lungs to the thoracic cavity should also be discussed in this exercise. The instructions for examination of the respiratory system of a cat are included in the *Laboratory Manual.* This exercise could be combined with exercises 38 and 39 for a laboratory period on respiration.

MATERIALS

1. Models and charts of the respiratory system
2. Fresh pluck (connected thoracic organs) of a sheep
3. Embalmed cat
4. Dissecting tray and dissecting instruments
5. Reference text
6. Colored pencils

KEY FOR LABELING EXERCISES

Figure 37.1 A sagittal section of the head showing the structures of the upper respiratory tract.

1. Nostril
2. Soft palate
3. Epiglottis
4. Glottis
5. Larynx
6. Superior nasal conchae
7. Middle nasal conchae
8. Inferior nasal conchae
9. Pharyngeal tonsils
10. Choana
11. Auditory (eustachian) tube
12. Palatine tonsil
13. Oropharynx
14. Lingual tonsil
15. Laryngopharynx

Figure 37.2 The larynx, trachea, and bronchial tree.

1. Epiglottis
2. Laryngeal prominence (Adam's apple)
3. Thyroid cartilage
4. Cricoid cartilage
5. Larynx
6. Trachea
7. Carina
8. Left primary bronchus
9. Secondary bronchi
10. Segmental bronchi
11. Terminal bronchioles
12. Glottis
13. True vocal chords
14. False vocal chords

Figure 37.3 An anterior view of the lower respiratory system.

1. Right superior lobe
2. Right middle lobe
3. Alveolar duct
4. Right inferior lobe
5. Alveoli
6. Left superior lobe
7. Cardiac notch
8. Left inferior lobe
9. Alveolar sac

Figure 37.4 A cross section of the thoracic cavity showing the mediastinum and pleural membranes.

1. Anterior mediastinum
2. Lung
3. Posterior mediastinum
4. Parietal pleura
5. Visceral pleura
6. Pleural cavity

Exercise 38 Measurements of Pulmonary Function

INTRODUCTION

This exercise is designed to introduce students to techniques to measure pulmonary function. Students should know that these techniques of spirometry are used by physicians to determine pulmonary function. It may also be helpful to discuss respiratory disorders, such as asthma, and the effects these disorders have on vital capacity and forced expiratory volume. This exercise could be combined with exercises 37 and 39 for a laboratory period on respiration.

MATERIALS

1. Collins, Inc., 9-liter respirometer
2. Disposable mouthpieces and nose clamp
3. Alternative equipment: Spirocomp™(Intelitool, Inc.) with Apple or IBM computer and wet 6L spirometer (Phipps and Bird)
4. Reference text

Exercise 39 Effects of Exercise on the Respiratory System

INTRODUCTION

This exercise is designed to examine the effects of exercise on respiration. A discussion of how CO_2 affects respiration would be very helpful, since exercise produces CO_2. This exercise could be combined with exercises 37 and 38 for a laboratory period on respiration.

MATERIALS

1. Spirometer (Collins 9-liter respirometer)
2. Disposable mouthpieces
3. Droppers, beakers, and straws
4. 0.10 *N* NaOH, phenolphthalein solution (saturated)

Exercise 40 Urinary System

INTRODUCTION

This exercise is designed to introduce students to the anatomy of the urinary system. This exercise could be combined with exercises 41, 42, and 43 for a laboratory period on the urinary system. Instructions for examining the urinary system of a cat are presented in the *Laboratory Manual* and may help students understand the structures of the urinary system.

MATERIALS

1. Fresh or preserved kidneys (sheep or pig)
2. Preserved cats
3. Dissection trays and instruments
4. Models and charts of the urinary system
5. Reference text
6. Atlas
7. Colored pencils

KEY TO LABELING EXERCISES

Figure 40.1 The urinary system.

1. Inferior vena cava
2. Kidney
3. Abdominal aorta
4. Ureter
5. Urinary bladder
6. Urethra

Figure 40.2 The internal structures of a kidney.

1. Renal pyramid
2. Renal cortex
3. Renal medulla
4. Minor calyx
5. Major calyx
6. Renal pelvis
7. Renal column
8. Renal papilla
9. Ureter

Figure 40.3 A simplified illustration of blood flow from a glomerulus to an efferent arteriole, the peritubular capillaries, and the venous drainage of the kidneys.

1. Glomerulus
2. Glomerular (Bowman's) capsule
3. Efferent arteriole
4. Afferent arteriole
5. Proximal convoluted tubule
6. Nephron loop (loop of Henle)
7. Distal convoluted tubule
8. Collecting duct

Figure 40.4 The vascular blood supply to the kidney.

1. Arcuate a.
2. Interlobular a.
3. Interlobar a.

Figure 40.5 An anterior view of the urinary bladder, ureters, and urethra.

1. Ureter
2. Trigone
3. Urethral orifice
4. Urethra
5. External urethral sphincter
6. Rugae of urinary bladder

Exercise 41 Renal Regulation of Fluid and Electrolyte Balance

INTRODUCTION

This exercise is designed to introduce students to renal physiology. The kidneys regulate fluid and electrolyte balance under the influence of ADH and aldosterone. In this exercise, students measure the effects of water loading and salt loading on urine concentration and specific gravity. This exercise could be combined with exercises 40, 42, and 43 for a laboratory period on the urinary system.

MATERIALS

1. Urine collection cups
2. Urinometers, droppers
3. pH paper (pH range 3-9), potassium chromate (20 g/dl), silver nitrate 2.9 g/dl)
4. NaCl crystals or salt tablets

Exercise 42 Renal Plasma Clearance of Urea

INTRODUCTION

This exercise is designed to introduce students to renal clearance of urea. In this exercise, students will measure renal plasma clearance rate and use the colorimeter to calculate the urea concentration of samples. This exercise could be combined with exercises 40, 41, and 43 for a laboratory period on the urinary system.

MATERIALS

1. Pipettes with mechanical pipettors (or Repipettes), mechanical microliter pipettes (capacity 20 μl), disposable tips
2. Colorimeter, cuvettes
3. BUN reagents and standard (Sclavo Diagnostics, available through Curtin-Matheson Scientific, Inc.)
4. Sterile lancets, 70% alcohol
5. File
6. Microhematocrit centrifuge and heparinized capillary tubes
7. Container for the disposal of blood-containing objects

Exercise 43 Clinical Examination of the Urine

INTRODUCTION

This exercise is designed to introduce students to techniques for examination of urine samples. Students will test urine for protein, ketone bodies, hemoglobin, bilirubin, and urine sediment. Remind the students that the tests they are performing are all tests performed in a clinical laboratory. This exercise could be combined with exercises 40, 41, and 42 for a laboratory period on the urinary system.

MATERIALS

1. Microscopes
2. Urine collection cups, test tubes, microscope slides, and cover slips
3. Albustix, Clinitest tablets, Ketostix, Hemastix, Ictotest tablets, or Multistix (all from Ames)
4. Sternheimer-Malbin stain
5. Centrifuge and centrifuge tubes
6. Transfer pipettes (droppers)

Exercise 44 Digestive System

INTRODUCTION

This exercise is designed to introduce students to the anatomy of the digestive system. Examination of histological slides of the digestive system will help students understand the function of the different sections and organs. Instructions for examination of the digestive system of a cat are given in the *Laboratory Manual*. This exercise could be combined with exercises 45, 46, and 47 for a complete laboratory period on the digestive system.

MATERIALS

1. Histological slides of specific regions of the GI tract and the accessory digestive organs
2. Models and charts of the digestive system
3. Tongue depressors, mirrors, and flashlights
4. Microscope
5. Reference text
6. Colored pencils
7. Preserved cats

KEY TO LABELING EXERCISES

Figure 44.1 The digestive system, including the GI tract and the accessory digestive organs.

1. Oral (buccal) cavity
2. Tongue
3. Teeth
4. Sublingual gland
5. Esophagus
6. Liver
7. Gallbladder
8. Large intestine
9. Small intestine
10. Parotid gland
11. Pharynx
12. Submandibular gland
13. Stomach
14. Pancreas

Figure 44.2 A midsagittal section of the abdominal cavity showing the peritoneum and various visceral organs.

1. Greater omentum
2. Lesser omentum
3. Mesentery
4. Visceral peritoneum
5. Parietal peritoneum

Figure 44.3 The structures of the oral cavity as seen through the oral orifice (the left side of the roof of the mouth is dissected to show the muscular soft palate).

1. Hard palate
2. Superior labial frenulum
3. Incisor teeth
4. Palatal rugae
5. Canine tooth
6. Premolar teeth
7. Molar tooth
8. Uvula
9. Palatine tonsil
10. Pharyngopalatine arch
11. Glossopalatine arch
12. Tongue
13. Lingual frenulum
14. Inferior labial frenulum

Figure 44.4 The dorsum of the tongue.

1. Vallate papillae
2. Fungiform papillae
3. Filiform papillae
4. Palatine tonsils

Figure 44.5 The structure of a tooth shown in a vertical section through a canine tooth.

1. Cusp
2. Enamel
3. Dentin
4. Cementum
5. Root
6. Neck
7. Gingiva
8. Alveolus

Figure 44.6 Salivary glands.

1. Parotid gland
2. Sublingual gland
3. Submandibular gland

Figure 44.7 A sagittal section of the facial region showing the oral cavity, nasal cavity, and pharynx.

1. Hard palate
2. Lips
3. Oral (buccal) cavity
4. Tongue
5. Vestibule
6. Soft palate
7. Uvula
8. Palatine tonsil
9. Oropharynx
10. Laryngopharynx

Figure 44.8 The major regions and structures of the stomach.

1. Esophagus
2. Longitudinal layer
3. Lesser curvature of stomach
4. Mucosa
5. Gastric rugae of mucosa
6. Pyloric sphincter
7. Pylorus of stomach
8. Greater curvature of stomach
9. Oblique layer
10. Circular layer
11. Body of stomach
12. Fundus of stomach
13. Cardia of stomach

Figure 44.9 The regions of the small intestine.

1. Duodenum
2. Duodenojejunal flexure
3. Jejunum
4. Ileum

Figure 44.10 The large intestine.

1. Hepatic flexure
2. Ascending colon
3. Ileocecal valve
4. Cecum
5. Appendix
6. Rectum
7. Transverse colon
8. Splenic flexure
9. Taeniae coli
10. Epiploic appendage
11. Descending colon
12. Haustrum
13. Sigmoid colon
14. Anal canal

Figure 44.11 Accessory digestive organs: the liver, gallbladder, and pancreas, and their associated structures.

1. Falciform ligament
2. Right lobe of liver
3. Quadrate lobe of liver
4. Gallbladder
5. Pancreatic duct
6. Left lobe of liver
7. Porta
8. Hepatic duct
9. Caudate lobe of liver
10. Cystic duct
11. Common bile duct
12. Tail of pancreas
13. Body of pancreas

Exercise 45 Digestion of Starch by Salivary Amylase

INTRODUCTION

This exercise is designed to demonstrate the activity of salivary amylase in the digestion of starch. Students will also see how pH and temperature affect enzyme activity. Reviewing principles of enzyme activity at this time would be very helpful to students. This exercise could be combined with exercises 44, 46, and 47 for a complete laboratory period on the digestive system.

MATERIALS

1. Water bath (set at 37°C), Bunsen burners, test tubes, test-tube clamp, graduated cylinders
2. Starch solution: dissolve 1.0 g/100 ml over heat
3. Iodine (Lugol's reagent): dissolve 1.0 g iodine and 2.0 g potassium iodide in 300 ml of water
4. Bendict's reagent: dissolve 50.0 g sodium carbonate, 85.0 g sodium citrate, and 8.5 g copper sulfate in 5.0 liters of water

Exercise 46 Digestion of Egg Albumin by Pepsin

INTRODUCTION

This exercise is designed to examine the action of pepsin, a digestive enzyme that breaks down protein. Since pepsin is the major enzyme produced in the stomach, students will benefit from examining its action. This exercise could be combined with exercises 44, 45, and 47 for a complete laboratory period on the digestive system.

MATERIALS

1. Water bath (set at 37°C), test tubes, droppers
2. Freezer or ice bath
3. Pepsin (5 g/100 ml), 2*N* HCl, 10*N* NaOH
4. White of hard-boiled eggs

Exercise 47 Digestion of Fat by Pancreatic Juice and Bile

INTRODUCTION

This exercise is designed to introduce students to the enzymatic activity of pancreatic juice and bile. Students will learn that bile acts to emulsify fats, while the pancreatic juice has the actual enzymatic activity to digest fats. This exercise could be combined with exercises 44, 45, and 46 for a complete laboratory period on the digestive system.

MATERIALS

1. Water bath (set at 37°C), test tubes, droppers
2. pH meter or short-range pH paper
3. Pancreatin solution (1g/dl), bile salts
4. Cream or vegetable oil

Exercise 48 Caloric Balance and Body Weight

INTRODUCTION

This exercise is designed to introduce students to methods of measuring caloric intake and expenditure, and the effects of caloric balance on body weight. This exercise requires students to measure their caloric intake and expenditure over 3 days, and then examine how this affected their body weight. It may be easiest to assign students to perform this exercise on their own, and then analyze their results during the laboratory period.

MATERIALS

1. Home scale or physicians height-weight scale
2. Calorie-counting guide such as the U.S. Department of Agriculture Handbook, cookbooks, or popular diet books

Exercise 49 Reproductive System

INTRODUCTION

This exercise is designed to introduce students to the anatomy of the male and female reproductive systems. An examination of histological slides of the reproductive organs may aid students in understanding the functions of these organs. This may be especially useful in examining the different stages of development of a follicle in the ovary. The instructions for examination of the reproductive system of a cat are presented in the *Laboratory Manual*. This exercise could be combined with exercises 50 and 51 for a complete laboratory period on the reproductive system.

MATERIALS

1. Microscopes
2. Prepared slides of the organs of the male and female reproductive systems—testis, epididymis, and ovary
3. Fresh or preserved reproductive organs from domestic animals
4. Models and charts of the male and female reproductive systems
5. Reference text
6. Colored pencils
7. Dissecting trays and instruments
8. Preserved cat

KEY TO LABELING EXERCISES

Figure 49.1 Organs of the male reproductive system: (*a*) a sagittal view; (*b*) a posterior view.

a.
1. Ductus (vas) deferens
2. Urethra
3. Penis
4. Glans penis
5. Prepuce
6. Seminal vesicle
7. Ejaculatory duct
8. Prostate
9. Bulbourethral gland
10. Epididymis
11. Testis
12. Scrotum

b.
1. Seminal vesicle
2. Ejaculatory duct
3. Bulbourethral gland
4. Epididymis
5. Testis
6. Penis
7. Urethra
8. Prepuce
9. Prostate
10. Ductus (vas) deferens
11. Glans penis

Figure 49.2 Structural features of the testis and epididymis (longitudinal view).
1. Head of epididymis
2. Body of epididymis
3. Tail of epididymis
4. Ductus (vas) deferens
5. Efferent ductules
6. Rete testis
7. Lobule containing seminiferous tubules
8. Septum
9. Tunica albuginea

Figure 49.3 The internal structure of the penis.
1. Corpora cavernosa penis
2. Corpus spongiosum penis
3. Dorsal vein
4. Urethra

Figure 49.4 The female reproductive organs (an anterior view).
1. Fimbriae
2. Follicle
3. Endometrium
4. Myometrium
5. Perimetrium
6. Fornix
7. Cervix
8. Vagina
9. Uterine (fallopian) tube
10. Body of uterus
11. Fundus
12. Ovary

Figure 49.5 The female reproductive organs (a sagittal view).
1. Fornix
2. Cervix
3. Vagina
4. Vaginal orifice
5. Labia minora
6. Labia majora
7. Uterine (fallopian) tube
8. Fimbriae
9. Ovary
10. Clitoris

Figure 49.6 The structure of the breast and mammary glands: (*a*) a sagittal section; (*b*) an anterior view partially sectioned.
1. Lactiferous duct
2. Mammary duct
3. Mammary glands
4. Nipple
5. Areola
6. Mammary duct

Figure 49.7 The external genitalia (vulva) of the female.
1. Clitoris
2. Labia majora
3. Labia minora
4. Mons pubis
5. Hymen
6. Vaginal orifice
7. Perineum

Exercise 50 Steroid Hormones

INTRODUCTION
This exercise is designed to introduce students to the steroid hormones secreted by the adrenal cortex and the gonads. In this exercise, students use thin-layer chromatography to compare the behavior of different steroid hormones. When the students are performing the thin-layer chromatography, they need to be sure that their steroid solution spots are above the level of the methanol when the TLC plates are placed in the chamber. They also need to mark the leading edge of their solution before drying the plates, or they will not be able to find it. This exercise could be combined with exercises 49 and 51 for a complete laboratory period on the reproductive system.

MATERIALS
1. Thin-layer plates (silica gel, F-254), chromatography developing chambers, capillary tubes
2. Driers (chromatography or hair driers), ultraviolet viewing box (short wavelength), rulers or spotting template (optional)
3. Steroid solutions in absolute methanol, 1.0 mg/ml of testosterone, of hydrocortisone, of cortisone, of corticosterone, and of deoxycorticosterone; 5 mg/ml of estradiol

4. Unknown steroid solution containing any two of the previous steroids
5. Developing solvent: 60 ml benzene plus 10 ml ethyl acetate plus 10 ml acetone, or a volume containing a comparable 6:1:1 solvent ratio

Exercise 51 Pregnancy Test

INTRODUCTION

This exercise is designed to introduce students to methods for determining pregnancy. Students actually perform a pregnancy test in the laboratory. This exercise could be combined with exercises 49 and 50 for a complete laboratory period on the reproductive system.

MATERIALS

1. Urine collection cup
2. Pregnancy kit (DAP test, Wampole test, or similar test)

Exercise 52 Patterns of Heredity

INTRODUCTION

This exercise is designed to introduce students to genetics and heredity. In this exercise, students will test themselves for PTC taste, discuss patterns of inheritance of ABO and Rh blood typing antigens, discuss sickle-cell anemia, and test for color blindness. All of these traits are heritable and students can use Punnett squares to determine their genotype for each of these traits.

MATERIALS

1. PTC paper
2. Sickle-Sol test tube (Dade)
3. Ishihara color blindness charts
4. Lancets and 70% alcohol

Answers to Laboratory Exercises

Laboratory Report 1 Body Organization and Terminology

A. Body Organization

1. cell
2. epithelial, connective, muscle, nervous
3. A tissue is a functional unit composed of cells and cell products that have similar specialized structures and functions. An organ is a structure in the body that is composed of more than one tissue.
4. A system consists of two or more organs that cooperate in the performance of particular functions.

B. Body Regions

head	axilla
manus	scapula
umbilicus	antebrachium
popliteal fossa	cervical region
palmar surface	plantar surface
lumbar region	thigh

C. Body Cavities

Cavity	*System*
dorsal	nervous
pericardial	circulatory
pleural	respiratory
abdominal	digestive
abdominal	digestive
dorsal	nervous

D. Descriptive Terminology

1.
a. superior	f. inferior
b. medial	g. posterior
c. distal	h. lateral
d. ventral	i. proximal
e. superficial	j. deep

2.
toward the head	away from the surface
toward the feet	toward the surface
toward the front	toward the trunk
toward the back	away from the trunk
toward the midline	pertaining to internal organs
away from the midline	pertaining to the body wall

Laboratory Report 2 Microscope and Metric System

A. Examination of the Microscope

1. to hold slide on stage
2. to provide highest magnification
3. to carry the microscope
4. to provide fine focus
5. to regulate the amount of light passing through the slide
6. to produce an image and magnify the image 10×

B. Use of the Microscope

1. First use the low-power objective. Bring this lens into its closest position to the slide, then focus away from the slide. When fine focus is achieved, switch to higher power and readjust with the fine focus. Take care not to allow the high-power lens to scrape the slide. Always put a microscope away with the low-power lens in the down position.
2. a. 4×
   b. 10×
   c. 45× or 43×
   d. 100×
3. a. 40×
   b. 100×
   c. 450× or 430×
   d. 1000×

C. Metric System and Dimensional Analysis

1. a. 1 g
   b. 0°C
   c. 1 L
2. 1. c 3. b
   2. a 4. d

D. Estimation of Microscopic Size

1. 400 μm
2. 270 μm
3. 120 μm
4. 270 μm

Laboratory Report 3 Homeostasis and Negative Feedback

A. Negative Feedback in a Constant-Temperature Water Bath

1. (Relates to data)
2. Homeostasis is the dynamic constancy of the internal environment. This constancy is maintained by negative feedback mechanisms, in which the effector acts to counter any deviations from a set point. Flow diagrams to answer this question are shown in chapter 1.

3. Flow diagrams similar to those in chapter 1 can be used. The diagrams should show that the heater turns on and the cooler turns off when the temperature falls and that the heater turns off and the cooler turns on when the temperature rises.

B. Negative Feedback Control of Pulse Rate

1. (Relates to data)
2. The up-and-down variation in successive pulse rate measurements suggests that pulse rate is under negative feedback control. A flow diagram can be drawn to show this. This diagram should include sympathetic nerve activity rising and parasympathetic activity declining when the pulse rate falls; the opposite changes occur when the pulse rate rises.

C. Normal Values

1. (Relates to data)
2. (Relates to data)
3. The normal range for a given measurement is obtained by taking measurements from a large sample of people who are believed to be normal for the measurement. There is always a range of values obtained, and this range, and its average, will vary with the group tested. This is why normal ranges for one population may be different from normal ranges for another population.

Laboratory Report 4 Measurement of Plasma Glucose, Protein, and Cholesterol

A. Introduction to the Colorimeter

1. directly proportional
2. Beer's law
3. The blank tube contains all of the reagents present in the other tubes except the test solution. Its function is to help set zero concentration equal to zero absorbance.
4. The graph should be a straight line because absorbance and concentration are directly proportional. Therefore, any deviation from a straight line is due to experimental error, which can be averaged by drawing a line through the scattering of points.

B. Measurement of Plasma Glucose Concentration

1. (Relates to data)
2. (Relates to data)
3. (Relates to data)
4. carbohydrate; monosaccharide
5. diabetes mellitus
6. insulin
7. When glucose levels are high, the liver and other organs can remove glucose from the blood. This is promoted by insulin. When blood glucose is low, the liver can secrete glucose into the blood.

C. Measurement of Plasma Cholesterol Concentration

1. (Relates to data)
2. (Relates to data)
3. (Relates to data)
4. lipid; steroid

5. atherosclerosis
6. All fats are lipids because all share the characteristic of being nonpolar and insoluble in water. Not all lipids are fats because steroids and phospholipids have different structures than triglycerides.

D. Measurement of Plasma Protein Concentration

1. (Relates to data)
2. (Relates to data)
3. (Relates to data)
4. (Relates to data)
5. amino acids, peptide
6. tertiary
7. liver
8. edema

Laboratory Report 5 Cell Structure and Cell Division

A. Structure of a Cell

1. centrioles
2. mitochondria
3. endoplasmic reticulum
4. nucleus
5. lysosome
6. ribosomes
7. cell (plasma) membrane

B. Cell Division

1. (1) d
   (2) a
   (3) c
   (4) b
2.

Mitosis	*Meiosis*
all cells	gonads
46	23
5	9

3. Mitosis produces two identical daughter cells for growth and repair. Meiosis is a special form of cell division by which gametes are formed for reproduction.

Laboratory Report 6 Genetic Control of Metabolism

1. a. DNA-directed RNA synthesis
   b. The synthesis of protein using the codons of RNA as a template
   c. A sequence of enzyme-catalyzed reactions in which the product of one enzyme becomes the substrate of the next
2. Since DNA determines RNA sequence, which then directs protein synthesis, a defect in the DNA will cause a different RNA to be made. Thus, a new protein will be synthesized that will not have the same chemical structure or properties. Therefore, metabolic pathways will be changed or blocked.

3. The diagram of phenylalanine metabolism is found in chapter 4, along with a discussion of how PKU, alkaptonuria, and albinism result from defective enzymatic steps in this pathway.

Laboratory Report 7 Diffusion, Osmosis, and Tonicity

A. Osmosis across a Synthetic Semipermeable Membrane

1. (Relates to data)
2. (Relates to data)
3. Osmosis is the passage of solvent (water) from a more dilute to a more concentrated solution through a membrane that is more permeable to water than to the solute.
4. Osmosis is passive because the water molecules move down their concentration gradient; metabolic energy is not required. The rate of osmosis depends on the difference in concentration of osmotically active solutes across the membrane, the surface area of membrane, and the temperature.

B. Osmosis across the Red Blood Cell Membrane

1. (Relates to data)
2. (Relates to data)
3. (Relates to data)
4. (Relates to data)
5. An isotonic solution has the same total solute concentration, osmolality, and osmotic pressure as the solution with which it is compared.
6. crenate
7. hypertonic
8.

NaCl	*Glucose*
0.133 M	0.200 M
133 mM	200 mM
266 mOsm	200 mOsm

   Osmosis will occur from the glucose to the NaCl solution because the NaCl solution is hypertonic to the glucose solution (assuming the membrane is not permeable to either solute). Since the NaCl solution is more concentrated than the glucose solution, solvent will move into the NaCl solution.
9. Seawater is hypertonic to the blood. Therefore, drinking seawater cannot dilute the blood and lower its osmolality. Since the receptors for thirst are stimulated by a high blood osmolality, drinking seawater cannot satisfy the sense of thirst.
10. Salting meat creates a hypertonic environment. Thus, when decomposing organisms (bacteria and fungi) come in contact with the salted meat, water will be drawn out of their cells, thus killing or inactivating them.

Laboratory Report 8 Histology

A. Epithelial Tissue

1. A tissue is an aggregate of similar cells and cellular products that performs specific functions. An organ is composed of a number of tissues and performs more complex functions.
2. Epithelial tissues may be classified as simple, if they are only one cell layer thick, or stratified, if they are two or more layers thick. Epithelial tissue may be further classified by the shape of its surface cells as squamous, cuboidal, or columnar.

B. Connective Tissue

1. Connective tissue is characterized by abundant amounts of extracellular material, or matrix. Unlike epithelial tissue, the cells of connective tissue are spread out from each other. Epithelial cells, in contrast, are tightly joined together, with very little matrix between them.
2. There are five types of connective tissues: (1) mesenchyme, (2) connective tissue proper, (3) cartilage, (4) bone, and (5) vascular (blood).
3. Hyaline cartilage — cartilages of trachea; fibrocartilage — intervertebral discs; elastic cartilage — pinna of ear.
4. Blood is a connective tissue because of its abundant extracellular material. The intercellular matrix of blood is called plasma. The blood cells are erythrocytes, leukocytes, and thrombocytes (platelets).

C. Muscular Tissue

1. Skeletal muscle — attached to the skeleton; cardiac muscle — the heart; smooth muscle — the walls of visceral organs and blood vessels.
2. Smooth muscle cells are long, spindle-shaped, and uninucleate. Cardiac muscle cells are striated, branched, and interconnected by intercalated discs. Skeletal muscle cells are long, fibrous, striated, and have multinucleate.

D. Nervous Tissue

1. Neurons and neuroglial cells are present in the nervous system. Neuroglia are more numerous. Neurons produce and conduct nerve impulses.
2. A cell process is a thin, cytoplasmic extension from the cell. The neuron has two types of processes. Dendrites are specialized for receiving stimulation, and axons are specialized for conducting impulses.

Laboratory Report 9 The Integumentary System

A. Layers of the Skin

1. (Relates to activity)
2. (Relates to activity)
3. Thick skin has more layers in the stratum corneum than thin skin. Also, thick skin has a stratum lucidum, which is absent in thin skin. Thick skin is found in the palms of the hand and soles of the feet, where it provides increased protection against abrasion. Thin skin is found everywhere else.
4. The stratum basale is composed of a single layer of columnarlike cells in contact with the dermis. These cells are constantly dividing mitotically and moving outward to renew the epidermis. The stratum corneum, with its keratin content, provides a toughened and water-resistant outer layer of the body.
5. A gradual exposure to sunlight promotes the increased production of melanin within the melanocytes, and hence tanning of the skin. The melanin granules help to absorb and disperse the sunlight. Excessive exposure to intense and continuous ultraviolet light can cause skin cancer.

B. Epidermal Derivatives

1. Drawing should appear something like figure 9.2 of lab manual.
2. Sebaceous glands are simple, branched glands that secrete an oily sebum into hair follicles. Sweat glands are coiled and tubular in shape and are located deeper in the dermis. These glands secrete perspiration onto the surface of the skin. Sweat glands are most numerous on the palms of the hands, soles of the feet, axillary and pubic regions, and the forehead.

3. Acne is an inflammatory condition of the sebaceous glands. It is affected by gonadal hormones and is therefore most common during puberty and adolescence.

Laboratory Report 10 Structure of Bone Tissue

1. *Long bones* are longer than they are wide and function as levers. Most of the bones of the upper and lower extremities are of this type. *Short bones* are somewhat cube-shaped and are found in confined spaces, where they transfer forces (wrist and ankle). *Flat bones* have a broad, dense surface for muscle attachment or protection of underlying organs (cranium, ribs, bones of the shoulder girdle). *Irregular bones* have varied shapes and have many surface markings for muscle attachment or articulation (vertebrae and certain bones of the skull).
2. The vascular supply of the bone is located in the central canal of each osteon. Nutrients and oxygen diffuse through the canaliculi to reach each osteocyte.
3.

Relationship	*Difference*
bone development	intramembranous — dense fibrous connective tissue; endochondral — hyaline cartilage
regions of long bones	diaphysis — shaft of bone; epiphysis — ends of bone
surface features of bones	fossa — flattened or shallow surface; foramen — a rounded opening
bone construction	compact — solid bone structure; spongy — latticelike bone structure
surface features of bones	tubercle — small, rounded process; trochanter — massive process found only in femur

Laboratory Report 11 Skeletal System: The Axial Skeleton

A. Skull

1. frontal, zygomatic, maxilla, lacrimal, ethmoid, palatine, and sphenoid bones
2. frontal, parietal, occipital, temporal, sphenoid, zygomatic, nasal, maxilla, mandible, and vomer
3.

Suture	*Articulating bones*
coronal	frontal bone with the two parietal bones
sagittal	left and right parietal bones
lambdoidal	occipital bone with two parietal bones
squamosal	parietal bone with the temporal bone

4. the vomer and the perpendicular plate of the ethmoid
5. the palatine processes of the maxillae and the palatine bones
6. the sphenoid, ethmoid, frontal, and maxillae bones

B. Hyoid Bone and Auditory Ossicles

1. The hyoid bone is located in the neck, just superior to the larynx. It is suspended from the stylohyoid processes of the skull by the stylohyoid ligaments. Several neck and tongue muscles attach to the hyoid bone.
2. The malleus, incus, and stapes are located in the middle ear cavity in the petrous part of the temporal bone. They transfer and amplify sound impulses through the middle ear.

C. Vertebral Column

Region	*Number of vertebrae*	*Diagnostic characteristics*
cervical	7	transverse foramina, bifurcating spinous processes
thoracic	12	facets, long spinous processes directed inferiorly
lumbar	5	thick bodies, blunt spinous processes
sacral	5 (fused)	fused spinous processes, dorsal sacral foramina, auricular surfaces
coccygeal	4–5 (fused)	triangular

D. Rib Cage

1. Seven pairs of true ribs each attach to the sternum by means of their own costal cartilages. There are five pairs of false ribs, two of which are floating (do not attach to the sternum at all).
2. The head of a rib articulates with a facet on the body of the thoracic vertebrae. The tubercle of a rib articulates with the fovea on the transverse process of the thoracic vertebrae.

Laboratory Report 12 Skeletal System: Appendicular Skeleton

A–D. Upper Extremity

1. The pectoral girdle is attached anteriorly to the axial skeleton by the flexible sternoclavicular joint. This type of attachment permits a wide range of movements of the upper extremity. The shoulder joints are supported primarily by muscle. Children, who have relatively weak muscles in this area, are thus vulnerable to shoulder dislocation.
2. A wedding ring is worn on the proximal phalanx of the fourth digit of the left hand.
3. a. a depressed area below the spine of the scapula
   b. the border of the scapula near the vertebral column
   c. a depressed area on the undersurface of the scapula
   d. the portion of the clavicle nearest the sternum
   e. a depressed area above the spine of the scapula
4. When the palm of the hand is up, the ulna and radius are parallel to each other. The radius will cross the ulna when the palm of the hand is in a downward position.
5. a. olecranon fossa of the humerus
   b. radial notch of ulna
   c. head of the radius
   d. coronoid process of the ulna

E–H. Lower Extremity

1. a. head of the femur
   b. condyles of the tibia
   c. talus
   d. patellar surface of the femur
2. a. patella
   b. phalanx
   c. scapula
   d. calcaneus
   e. medial epicondyle of the humerus
   f. os coxa

g. clavicle
h. anterior crest of the tibia
i. medial malleolus of tibia and lateral malleolus of fibula
j. head of metacarpal bone
k. scaphoid, cuneiform

3. Refer to text radiographs.

Laboratory Report 13 Articulations

A. Joints

1. False. Synarthrotic joints are rigid and immovable because the articulating bones are tightly connected by either fibrous tissue or cartilage.
2. a. lubricates and protects joints and associated structures
   b. surrounds joints and contains synovial fluid
   c. directs joint movement and cushions joint
   d. facilitates joint movement
   e. supports the bones of a joint and attaches bone to bone
   f. lining of the joint capsule; produces synovial fluid
   g. near joints; provides cushioning
3. a. femur, tibia, patella
   b. humerus, ulna, radius
   c. ilium, ischium, pubis, femur
   d. ulna, radius, proximal carpal bones
   e. tibia, fibula, calcaneus
   f. clavicle, scapula, humerus
4. The skull of a newborn must be flexible to facilitate parturition and the growth of the brain.
5. a. An interosseous ligament is a sheet of connective tissue that binds parallel bones.
   b. Hyaline cartilage is a type of cartilage. Articular cartilage, costal cartilage, and menisci are made of hyaline cartilage.
   c. Intervertebral discs separate and provide movability to vertebrae.
   d. A symphysis is a type of cartilaginous joint that permits slight movement.

B. Movements at Synovial Joints

1. The shoulder joint is an extremely mobile ball-and-socket joint designed for movement and muscle attachment; it cannot withstand large amounts of stress. The hip joint is a ball-and-socket joint that bears the weight of the body and functions in locomotion. Thus, it is much stronger and more stable than the shoulder joint.
2.

	Knee	*Elbow*
Size	larger	smaller
Shape	hinge	complex hinge
No. of bones	three	three
Movement	flexion, extension	flexion, extension, gliding, rotation

Laboratory Report 14 Neural Control of Skeletal Muscle Contraction

1. sarcomere
2. myosin; actin
3. Length of the A band does not change; I and H bands shorten during contraction. Conclusion: length of thin and thick filaments does not change during contraction.
4. Ca^{++} couples electrical excitation to contraction. This occurs because electrical excitation stimulates the release of Ca^{++} from the sarcoplasmic reticulum, and Ca^{++}, in turn, combines with troponin to activate the contraction cycle of the cross-bridges.
5. A threshold is the minimum stimulus that will produce a given response—in this case, measurable contraction. The threshold is lower when the nerve is stimulated because a lower voltage is required to activate the thinner nerve fibers compared to the thicker muscle. When a given nerve axon is stimulated, it can stimulate all of the muscle fibers in its motor unit to contract.

Laboratory Report 15 Summation, Tetanus, and Fatigue

A. Summation, Tetanus, and Fatigue in Frog Gastrocnemius Muscle

1. (Relates to data)
2. (Relates to data)
3. Summation of twitches was produced in this exercise by stimulating the muscle with successive shocks. Each successive shock produced a twitch that began before the muscle could relax from the previous twitch, so that the extent of shortening of the muscle was increased by the summation process. Variations in the strength of muscle contraction are produced by a similar mechanism, in which increasing the number of muscle fibers stimulated increases the summation of their responses, and this produces a stronger contraction.
4. Muscle fatigue is usually caused by accumulation of lactic acid, which interferes with excitation-contraction coupling. If a muscle fiber ran out of ATP, the fiber would remain in a contracted state analogous to rigor mortis.

B. Twitch, Summation, and Tetanus in Human Muscle

1. The finger twitched in response to separate shocks, and as the shocks occurred more rapidly, the twitches summated to eventually produce a tetanus. (Relates to data)
2. Normal muscular movements must also be a result of electrical stimulation occurring in the body.
3. Sustained contractions in vitro were produced by delivering shocks to the muscle in rapid succession. Sustained contractions in vivo are produced by rapid asynchronous activation of motor neurons and their motor units.

Laboratory Report 16 Muscles of the Head and Neck

1. orbicularis oris
   frontalis
   orbicularis oculi
   orbicularis oculi
   zygomaticus
   depressor angularis
2. masseter
3. digastric
4. sternocleidomastoid
5. styloglossus
6. medial pterygoid

Laboratory Report 17 Muscles of the Pectoral Girdle and Upper Extremity

A and B. Muscles That Act on the Pectoral Girdle and Muscles That Move the Humerus

1. axial
2. scapula
3. latissimus dorsi
4. a. push-ups, bench press
   b. lateral raises (abduction), military press
   c. push-ups, bench press
   d. pull-ups, rowing, swimming
5. (Relates to activity)

C and D. Muscles That Act on the Forearm and Muscles That Move the Wrist, Hand, and Fingers

1. biceps brachii, brachialis, and brachioradialis
2. pronator teres, flexor carpi radialis, palmaris longus, flexor carpi ulnaris, flexor carpi radialis, and superficial digital flexor
3. flexor carpi radialis and flexor carpi ulnaris

Laboratory Report 18 Muscles of the Trunk and Lower Extremity

A. Muscles of the Trunk

1. Exercises such as sit-ups and leg-lifts can help strengthen the abdominal muscles.
2. The sartorius and adductor longus provide two boundaries of the femoral triangle (the third boundary is the inguinal ligament). This area is of clinical importance because it is a pressure point for the femoral artery, and it is a common site of hernias through the femoral ring of the inguinal ligament.

B and C. Muscles of the Hip and Thigh

1. The advantages are (1) division of labor, (2) greater range of motion, and (3) more precise movement.
2. The adductor muscles assist in stabilizing the hip joint because of their sites of origin and insertion. All of these muscles originate on either the pubic or ischial regions of the os coxae and insert on the upper femur or upper tibia. This structural arrangement gives additional strength and support to the hip region.

D. Muscles of the Leg

1. *Anteriorly:* tibialis anterior, extensor hallucis longus, peroneus tertius, extensor digitorum longus
   Laterally: peroneus longus, peroneus brevis
   Posteriorly: tendo calcaneus of the gastrocnemius and soleus, flexor digitorum longus, flexor hallucis longus, and tibialis posterior
2. *Lateral malleolus:* peroneus longus and peroneus brevis
   Medial malleolus: flexor hallucis longus, flexor digitorum longus, and tibialis posterior
3. The popliteal fossa is the posterior region of the knee. The popliteal artery, popliteal vein, tibial nerve, and peroneal nerve all pass through the popliteal fossa.

General Questions

Description	*Muscles*
Hamstrings	biceps femoris, semitendinosus, semimembranosus
Lower back muscle	quadratus lumborum, lower portion of sacrospinalis
Abdominal "strap" muscle	rectus abdominous
Tailor's muscle	sartorius
Calf muscle	gastrocnemius, soleus
Adductor muscles	gracilis, pectineus, adductor longus, adductor brevis, adductor magnus
Abdominal compression	external oblique, internal oblique, transverse abdominous, rectus abdominis

Laboratory Report 19 Cat Musculature

A–C. Muscles of the Neck, Shoulder, and Back Regions

1. The cutaneous maximus moves the skin of the cat. Humans do not need this exaggerated movement of the skin.
2. clavotrepezius styloglossus
   temporalis hypoglossus
3. rhomboideus major, rhomboideus minor, levator scapulae ventralis, serratus ventralis, and pectoralis minor
4. deep: supraspinatus, infraspinatus, teres major, teres minor, subscapularis; superficial: acromiodeltoid, spinodeltoid

D and E. Muscles of the Thoracic and Abdominal Regions

1. The levator scapulae ventralis, pectoantebrachialis, and xiphihumeralis muscles are present in the cat because it is a quadruped and this has different requirements than the bipedal human.
2. The levator scapulae originates on the last five cervical vertebrae and insert on the medial surface of the scapula. Its action is to draw the scapula cranioventrad. The levator scapulae ventralis originates on the occipital bone and the atlas (C1) and inserts on the metacromion process. Its action is to draw the scapula craniad.
3. The force of gravity is exerted differently on the abdomen of a quadruped such as a cat than on the abdomen of a bipedal human. The abdominal muscles of a cat must be more developed than those of a human because they support the abdominal organs. In a human, the abdominal organs are supported more by the pelvic architecture and mesenteric sites of attachment to the body cavity.

F. Muscles of the Brachium

1. epitrochlearis, triceps brachii, and anconeus
2. The triceps brachii extends the forelimbs against the force of gravity during locomotion, whereas the biceps brachii only flexes the forelimbs so that they are elevated during the swing phase of the locomotor cycle.
3. The larger number of forearm muscles provide more precision in movements of the cat's paw. Their mass is less because they do not need to produce as much force as the muscles of the brachium.

G. Muscles of the Hip and Thigh Regions

1. The massive sartorius of the cat is a major extensor muscle of the knee joint. It is an important synergist to the quadriceps femoris. In the human, the sartorius is a thin, straplike muscle that wraps from lateral to medial across the anterior surface of the thigh. Its major actions in humans are to flex the leg and thigh and to rotate the leg medially.
2. Hind limb muscles of a cat that are not present in humans are the tenuissimus and caudofemoralis. The hind limb muscle of a human that is not present in the cat is the adductor magnus.

Laboratory Report 20 Brain and Cranial Nerves

1. Refer to figure 20.2 in the lab manual.
2. a. metencephalon
   b. myelencephalon
   c. telencephalon
   d. diencephalon
3. a. trigeminal, abducens, facial, and vestibulocochlear
   b. glossopharyngeal, vagus, accessory, hypoglossal, and vestibulocochlear
   c. oculomotor, trochlear
4. The arteries that contribute to the cerebral arterial circle are the internal carotid arteries, which form the middle cerebral arteries, and the vertebral arteries, which form the basilar artery. The basilar artery, in turn, forms the posterior cerebral arteries. Communicating arteries complete the circle. The significance of this circle is that it provides collateral circulation so that obstruction in the flow of blood in one vessel will not completely prevent blood from reaching the different areas of the brain.
5. a. facial (motor portion) nerve
   b. vestibular branch of the vestibulocochlear nerve
   c. oculomotor nerve
   d. glossopharyngeal nerve
   e. accessory nerve
   f. ophthalmic branch of the trigeminal nerve
   g. oculomotor nerve
   h. facial (sensory portion) nerve
   i. oculomotor nerve

6.

Location	*Function*
diencephalon	relay center, especially for pain
diencephalon	decussation of tracts for optic fibers
diencephalon	major endocrine gland
metencephalon	relay center and origin for some cranial nerves
myelencephalon	relay center and autonomic control center
metencephalon	motor tracts within cerebellum
diencephalon	may have some role in regulation of puberty
entire CNS	protection
mesencephalon	auditory reflexes

7. The first and second (lateral) ventricles are located within the cerebral hemispheres. The third ventricle is near the thalamus, and the fourth ventricle is at the base of the cerebellum. Cerebrospinal fluid is produced in the choroid plexuses. It circulates slowly by the action of ciliated ependymal cells and drains into the venous sinuses at the arachnoid villi.

Laboratory Report 21 Spinal Cord, Spinal Nerves, and Spinal Reflexes

A. Spinal Cord

1. The central nervous system includes the brain and spinal cord. The neurons in the CNS are association neurons. The peripheral nervous system includes sensory and motor neurons and their associated ganglia.
2. Refer to figure 21.2 in the lab manual.
3. "Mixed" nerves contain both motor and sensory neurons and therefore convey impulses both to and from the spinal cord.
4. a. a collection of axons in the PNS
   b. a grouping of cell bodies in the PNS
   c. the "horse's tail" appearance of spinal nerves descending from the termination of the spinal cord inferiorly within the filum terminale
   d. the extension of the meninges of the spinal cord inferior to the termination of the spinal cord

B. Structure of the Reflex Arc

1. (1) b
   (2) d
   (3) a
   (4) c

C and D. Spinal Nerve Stretch Reflexes and Cutaneous Reflex

1. Striking the patellar ligament causes the quadriceps femoris muscles to stretch. When the spindles within these muscles are stretched, action potentials are stimulated in the sensory neurons. These action potentials are conducted by sensory neurons into the gray matter of the spinal cord, where the sensory neurons synapse with motor neurons. Action potentials are produced in the motor neurons, and these action potentials are conducted to the axon endings, which release ACh and stimulate contraction of the muscle.
2. A given stretch reflex involves the synapse between sensory and motor neurons at only one level of the spinal cord. In the Babinski reflex, the sensory information ascends from the lumbar region of the spinal cord to the brain, and motor pathways that descend from the brain to the lumbar region of the spinal cord are activated. Damage to the spinal cord at any level can therefore interrupt this flow of impulses and produce an abnormal Babinski reflex.

E. Referred Pain

1. The pain was felt in the fingers, in this exercise, because the sensory neurons in the median ulnar nerve are normally stimulated in this region and the brain interprets impulses in this nerve as arising from the normal site of stimulation.
2. Deep visceral pain is poorly localized, but damage to visceral organs may cause pain in characteristic somatic locations, and by this means, the nature of the damage may be more easily diagnosed. Examples include pain in the left arm and substernal areas caused by myocardial ischemia and subscapular pain caused by gallstones.
3. The sensory organs transduce different forms of energy into nerve impulses, which are transmitted to the brain. The brain interprets impulses arriving along different neural pathways as particular sensations in particular parts of the body. The fact that we perceive with the brain is shown by the phantom limb phenomenon, in which the brain is "tricked" by the arrival of impulses along nerves that normally serve the missing limb and, as a result, pain is perceived in the missing limb.

Laboratory Report 22 Cutaneous Receptors

A and B. Structure of the Cutaneous Receptors, and Mapping the Temperature and Touch Receptors of the Skin

1. (Relates to activity)
2. You can conclude that there are different receptors for hot, cold, and touch, which are located in different places in the skin. These receptors are specialized dendritic endings of sensory neurons.

C. Two-Point Touch Threshold

1. (Relates to data)
2. The punctate distribution of cutaneous receptors refers to the fact that these receptors are located at specific points in the skin. This is illustrated by the fact that a thin object, such as a bristle or the point of a caliper, can only be felt at specific points on the skin and not at other locations.
3. The picture is a map of the sensory and motor cortex. Somatesthetic sensations from a given part of the body project to the area of sensory cortex indicated by the map. The area of the motor cortex represented by an image of a body region controls muscles in that region. These maps were obtained by electrically stimulating the cerebral cortex of awake patients during brain surgery.

D. Adaptation of Temperature Receptors

1. The hand that was previously in warm water felt colder, while the hand that was previously in cold water felt warmer. This difference in perception was due to the fact that the receptors for cold in one hand and those for warmth in the other hand experienced sensory adaptation in the first water bath.
2. Sensory adaptation refers to the decline in the intensity of a sensation over time with continued stimulation of the receptor. Senses of touch and smell adapt quickly; the sense of pain adapts slowly, if at all.

Laboratory Report 23 Eyes and Vision

1. a. iris
   b. fovea centralis
   c. cornea
   d. blind spot
2.

Innervation	*Function*
oculomotor	elevates the upper eyelid
parasympathetic and sympathetic	regulates the amount of light that enters the pupil
abducens	rotates eye away from midline
oculomotor	rotates eye toward midline
oculomotor	rotates eye upward and toward midline
oculomotor	rotates eye downward and toward midline
trochlear	rotates eye downward and away from midline
oculomotor	rotates eye upward and away from midline

3. (1) b
   (2) d
   (3) e
   (4) a
   (5) c
4. a. Visual acuity is the ability of the eye to resolve points in a figure, which is related to the clarity of vision.
   b. Accommodation is the ability of the eye to focus the image of an object on the retina when the object is different distances from the eye.
   c. Convergence is overlapping of the medial regions of the visual field of both eyes.
   d. Nystagmus is uncontrolled and grossly apparent oscillations of the eyes, where they move in one direction relatively slowly and are forced back to a forward position more rapidly.
5. The iris controls the aperture of the pupil. Circularly arranged muscles in the iris cause constriction of the pupil, and radial muscles cause dilation of the pupil.
6. Light passes through the cornea, aqueous humor, lens, vitreous body, ganglion cells, bipolar cells, and finally to the photoreceptors. Light is refracted by the cornea and lens.
7. A person with myopia has an abnormally long eyeball, so that the focus of an image is in front of the retina. When the object is moved closer to the eye, the focus moves back to the retina and produces a sharper image. A person with normal vision, in contrast, must increase the curvature of the lens to prevent the focus from moving behind the retina as the object is brought closer to the eye.
8. Rods provide greater visual sensitivity than cones, because rods can respond to low light intensity. This sensitivity comes from the fact that the all-trans form is more sensitive than the 11-cis form of retinaldehyde, but only 11-cis-retinaldehyde is associated with opsin. Dissociation of opsin from retinaldehyde causes an action potential and this is easily achieved because the dissociated form is more sensitive than the associated form. Cones provide greater visual acuity than rods, because cones have a lower degree of convergence. Since each cone in the fovea has a direct input to a ganglion neuron, images can be very precise. The fovea has the greatest concentration of cones, and thus it has the greatest acuity.
9. Light entering the eye creates action potentials in the optic nerves. These action potentials travel to the brain. Once these signals reach the brain they are processed and an image is created. For this reason you see with your brain and not with your eyes.
10. Carotene is a precursor to vitamin A and vitamin A is a precursor to retinaldehyde. Supplying the body with carotene can therefore increase the amount of retinaldehyde in the rods. This will increase the sensitivity of the eye and improve night vision.

Laboratory Report 24 Ears and Hearing

A. Anatomy of the Ear

1. 10 Cochlear duct
   13 Cochlear nerve
   2 External auditory canal
   12 Hair cells
   5 Incus
   4 Malleus
   11 Spiral organ (organ of Corti)
   7 Oval window
   1 Auricle
   9 Scala tympani
   8 Scala vestibuli
   6 Stapes
   3 Tympanic membrane
2. See figure 24.2 in the lab manual. The scala tympani and scala vestibuli contain perilymph, and the cochlear duct contains endolymph.

B. Conduction of Sound Waves through Bone: Rinne and Weber's Tests

1. Sound waves in air cause vibrations of the tympanic membrane, which cause movements of the middle ear ossicles. As the stapes pushes against the oval window, compression waves of endolymph are set up and cause vibrations of the basilar and vestibular membranes. As the hair cell processes press against the overhanging tectorial membrane, they are bent, and this bending stimulates the production of nerve impulses.
2. The pitch of a sound determines the pattern of vibration of the basilar membrane. Low pitches cause the basilar membrane to vibrate as a unit, whereas higher pitches cause maximum vibration of the basilar membrane closer to its base. Hair cells in different regions of the basilar membrane are thus excited in accordance with the pitch of the sound. The loudness of a sound is related to the amplitude with which the basilar membrane is displaced and thus is related to the extent of activation of the hair cells in a given region of the membrane. Nerve impulses will thus be produced with greater frequency in the nerve fibers serving the stimulated sensory cells.
3. If a person with otosclerosis performed the Rinne test, he or she would hear the sound when the tuning fork was placed against the mastoid process of the temporal bone but not when the tuning fork was placed outside the ear. This is because sound waves can stimulate the inner ear by conduction through bone (bypassing the middle ear) but cannot be transmitted by the middle ear ossicles. In Weber's test the sound will appear loudest in the ear with otosclerosis, just as it does in a person with normal hearing who plugs one ear. This is because the brain can pay more attention to sounds coming to the ear by bone conduction when distracting sounds are eliminated.

Laboratory Report 25 Taste

1. (Relates to activity)
2. a. the tip of the tongue
   b. the tip and edge of the tongue
   c. the back of the tongue
   d. the lateral edges of the tongue
3. Since the glossopharyngeal nerve serves the posterior third of the tongue, damage to this nerve would most reduce the sensation of bitter taste. Destruction of the facial nerve would most reduce the sensation of sweet, salty, and sour tastes because the facial nerve innervates the anterior two-thirds of the tongue where sweet, salty, and sour tastes are concentrated.

A. Pituitary Gland

1. Pituitary: hypophysis
   Anterior pituitary: adenohypophysis
   Posterior pituitary: neurohypophysis
2. The anterior pituitary is derived from epithelial tissue (Rathke's pouch) and produces and secretes hormones. It is thus very metabolically active and stains intensely. The posterior pituitary is derived from neural tissue and does not synthesize the hormones it secretes. It is thus not very metabolically active and does not stain very intensely. The functional significance is that hormones are produced in the anterior portion of the pituitary; hence its glandular appearance. The posterior portion does not produce hormones and therefore does not have a glandular appearance.
3. The hypothalamus regulates the secretion of the posterior pituitary by means of nerve impulses arriving on the hypothalamo-hypophyseal tract. The hypothalamus regulates the secretion of the anterior pituitary by secreting releasing and inhibiting hormones into the hypothalamo-hypophyseal portal system.

B. Thyroid and Parathyroid Glands

1. Tetraiodothyronine (thyroxine) and triiodothyronine
2. The major function of the thyroid in an adult is to regulate the basal metabolic rate and to regulate calcium levels. The parathyroids regulate calcium balance.

C and D. Pancreatic Islets and Adrenal Glands

1. Exocrine glands secrete the products into ducts, whereas endocrine glands secrete hormones into the blood. The exocrine acini of the pancreas secrete pancreatic juice into the pancreatic duct, whereas the pancreatic islets secrete insulin and glucagon into the blood.
2. Insulin promotes the anabolism of glycogen and fat as well as promoting the entry of glucose into tissue cells. Glucagon promotes the breakdown of glycogen to glucose in the liver.
3. Adrenal cortex: mineralocorticoids, glucocorticoids, and sex steroids. Adrenal medulla: epinephrine and lesser amounts of norepinephrine.
4. The adrenal cortex is derived from mesoderm, whereas the adrenal medulla is derived from neural crest, just as are the sympathetic ganglia. The adrenal medulla is thus innervated by preganglionic sympathetic nerve fibers, whereas the adrenal cortex is not. The secretions of the adrenal cortex are regulated by ACTH secreted by the anterior pituitary gland.

E and F. Ovaries and Testes

1. An ovarian follicle contains an inner wall called a theca interna, granulosa cells, and an ovum. The theca interna produces testosterone, which is changed by granulosa cells into estradiol, which is secreted.
2. The two compartments of the testes are the seminiferous tubules and the interstitial cells. The seminiferous tubules produce sperm, whereas the interstitial cells produce testosterone. Since a vasectomy interferes with the transport of sperm, a vasectomy will block sperm transport and abolish fertility but will have no effect on testosterone secretion.

G. Pineal Gland, Placenta, and Thymus

1. estrogen, progesterone, chorionic gonadotropin, chorionic somatomammotropin
2. brain, intestinal tract, pancreas, liver, kidney, heart, ovary, testis
3. The pineal gland is located in the roof of the third ventricle; the thymus is located deep to the manubrium. The pineal gland may function in regulating the reproductive system. The thymus processes T cells and helps to regulate the immune system.

Laboratory Report 27 Red Blood Cells and Oxygen Transport

1. (Relates to data)
2. (Relates to data)
3. (Relates to data)
4. (Relates to data)
5. (Relates to data)
6. 4, 4
7. erythropoietin
8. kidneys
9. bilirubin
10. jaundice
11. hematocrit
12. oxyhemoglobin
13. methemoglobin
14. carboxyhemoglobin
15. Anemia is a condition characterized by an abnormally low red blood cell count and/or hemoglobin concentration. It may be caused by a high rate of red blood cell destruction or insufficient red blood cell production. The latter situation may be due to conditions such as iron deficiency or deficiency of vitamin B_{12}. This condition is dangerous because of low O_2 capacity.
16. A rapid rate of red blood destruction results in the liberation of excessive amounts of heme from hemoglobin. These free heme molecules are converted into bilirubin, which circulates in the blood. If the liver cannot get rid of this bilirubin by conjugating it and excreting it in the bile, then the blood concentration of bilirubin can rise to a sufficient level to produce jaundice. Babies often develop jaundice because their livers are not fully functional at the time of birth.

Laboratory Report 28 Total and Differential White Blood Cell Counts

A. Total White Blood Cell Count

1. (Relates to data)
2. (Relates to data)

B. Differential White Blood Cell Count

1. (Relates to data)
2. (Relates to data)
3. a. neutrophils
   b. lymphocytes
   c. eosinophils
   d. basophils
4. B; T
5. diapedesis
6. neutrophil

7. The combination of antibodies with antigens on the cell surface of the pathogen stimulates phagocytosis. This occurs directly and indirectly via the activation of complement proteins. Some of the complement proteins attract phagocytic cells to the site of the infection, keep these cells at the site, and stimulate the activity of the phagocytic cells.
8. T lymphocytes either come from or had an ancestor that came from the thymus. B cells come from the bone marrow. T cells provide cell-mediated immunity; some secrete lymphokines, whereas others either help or suppress the immune response. B cells can be transformed into antibody-secreting plasma cells, which provide humoral immunity.
9. A clone of lymphocytes is a large population of genetically identical cells that are each able to respond specifically to a particular antigen. Such a clone is produced by prior exposure to the antigen, which stimulates cells with the proper receptor molecule to divide by mitosis numerous times and produce the clone.
10. Exposure to a pathogen with reduced virulence that has the same antigenicity as the fully virulent form allows the immune system to become sensitized to those antigens. Clones of lymphocytes are produced, so that when the person is exposed to the virulent pathogen, the immune system mounts a secondary rather than a primary response.
11. The advantages of passive immunizations are that protection is rapid and does not require prior exposure to sensitize the immune system. The disadvantages of passive immunizations are that the person does not develop immunity to subsequent exposure to the same pathogen and that injections of serum from another animal into a human can cause an immune reaction against the antigens present in the antiserum. The advantages of active immunity include the fact that immunity to subsequent exposures is developed. The main disadvantage is that it takes longer for the individual to respond.

Laboratory Report 29 Blood Types

1. (Relates to data)
2. (Relates to data)
3. (Relates to data)
4. (Relates to data)
5.

	antigens present	*antigens not present*
a.	A	B, Rh
b.	Rh	A, B
c.	A, B	Rh

6. A person with A negative blood has antibodies against B antigens and against Rh antigens. Therefore the antibodies would attack the recipients B and Rh antigens and cause agglutination.
7. For hemolytic disease of the newborn to occur, there must be an Rh+ father, Rh− mother, and Rh+ baby. At delivery the mothers's blood may be exposed to the Rh antigen from the baby and develop antibodies against it. If a second child is Rh+, antibodies from the mother may cross the placenta and destroy the fetal red blood cells. The development of maternal antibodies against the Rh factor may be prevented by administration of Rh antibodies (RHOgam) shortly after labor. These antibodies destroy any fetal red blood cells which may have entered the mothers blood supply before the mother can produce antibodies against them.
8. The blood types in this case can neither prove nor disprove her claim, because the man who is type A could have either of two genotypes—AA or AO. If he has the AA genotype, he cannot have fathered a type O child, but if he has the AO genotype, there is a 50% chance that he could have fathered a type O child.

Laboratory Report 30 Heart and Arteries

A and B. Heart, Dissection of Mammalian Heart

1. *Right Side* — *Left Side*

Right Side	*Left Side*
three cusps	two cusps
moderate	very thick
low oxygen	high oxygen
three	four

2. Blood passes through the superior vena cava, inferior vena cava, or coronary sinus to the right atrium, right atrioventricular valve, right ventricle, pulmonary valve, pulmonary trunk, pulmonary arteries, lungs, pulmonary veins, left atrium, left atrioventricular valve, left ventricle, aortic valve, and ascending aorta.
3. A cardiac impulse passes through the sinoatrial (SA) node, atria, atrioventricular (AV) node, atrioventricular bundle, conduction myofibrils, and ventricles.

C. Blood Vessels

1. The pulmonary arteries (vessles that carry blood away from the heart) carry deoxygenated blood from the right ventricle to the lungs. The pulmonary veins (vessels that carry blood towards the heart) carry oxygenated blood from the lungs to the left atrium.
2. *Artery* — *Vein*

Artery	*Vein*
smaller than veins	larger than arteries
little variation	tremendous variation
away from the heart	to the heart
thick walls	thin walls
deep	superficial and deep

D. Principal Arteries of the Body

1. a. coronary arteries
   b. renal artery
   c. external carotid artery
   d. internal iliac artery
   e. phrenic artery
   f. vertebral arteries and internal carotid arteries
   g. ovarian artery
   h. left gastric and splenic arteries
   i. inferior mesenteric artery
2. a. radial artery
   b. celiac artery
   c. left common carotid artery
   d. popliteal artery
   e. brachiocephalic artery
   f. brachial artery
   g. femoral artery
3. Those not symmetrical are the brachiocephalic trunk, aorta, basilar artery, celiac trunk, hepatic artery, left gastric artery, splenic artery, superior mesenteric artery, and inferior mesenteric artery.

Laboratory Report 31 Veins, Lymphatics, and Fetal Circulation

A. Principal Veins of the Body

1. The path includes the median cubital vein, basilic vein, axillary vein, subclavian vein, brachiocephalic vein, superior vena cava, right atrium, right atrioventricular valve, right ventricle, pulmonary valve, pulmonary trunk, pulmonary artery, lungs, pulmonary vein, left atrium, left atrioventricular valve, left ventricle, aortic valve, ascending aorta, brachiocephalic trunk*, right common carotid artery*, right internal carotid artery*, anterior and middle cerebral arteries*, and brain. The steps with the asterisk(*)

may be replaced as follows: left common carotid artery, left internal carotid artery, anterior and middle cerebral arteries, and brain.

2. A portal system is a vascular pattern in which two capillary beds are in series with each other; that is, one lies downstream from the other. The two capillary beds are connected by veins, and the second is drained by veins into the general circulation. Such a pattern exists to deliver molecules from one organ (where the first capillary bed is located) to another organ (where the second capillary bed is located).
3. a. ovarian (gonadal) vein
   b. internal jugular vein
   c. deep femoral vein, great saphenous vein
   d. hepatic vein
   e. inferior mesenteric vein
   f. ulnar vein, radial vein, cephalic vein, basilic vein
   g. lumbar vein, azygos vein
   h. phrenic vein
   i. cystic vein
   j. pancreatic vein
   k. renal vein
   l. left gastric vein, left gastroepiploic vein, right gastric vein, right gastroepiploic vein

B. Fetal Circulation

1. The majority of the blood flowing through the fetal heart is shunted through the foramen ovale so that it does not pass into the right ventricle. The blood is shunted away from the pulmonary circulation, because oxygen-carbon dioxide exchange takes place at the placenta, not the lungs.
2. umbilical vein, umbilical arteries, ductus venosus, foramen ovale, and ductus arteriosus
3. Congenital heart disorders result from abnormalities in embryonic development and may be attributed to heredity, diet of the pregnant mother, or viral infections during pregnancy. Examples include atrial and ventricular septal defects, pulmonary stenosis, and tetralogy of Fallot. Acquired heart disease may occur suddenly or gradually during the individual's lifetime. Examples include inadequate coronary blood supply, atherosclerosis, conduction disturbances, bacterial endocarditis, myocardial disease, and pericardial disease.

C. Lymphatic System

1. This usually indicates that the person has an infection in the body. It occasionally may indicate cancer of the thyroid, which has metastasized to the cervical lymph nodes.
2. The thymus and the spleen are lymphoid organs because they contain phagocytic reticular tissue and also contain centers for lymphocyte production. They differ in size, structure, and immune function.
3. Metastasized cancer of the breast would first afflict the localized lymph nodes within the mammary and adipose tissue. It would then secondarily spread to the axillary lymph nodes.

Laboratory Report 32 Effects of Drugs on the Frog Heart

1. (Relates to data)
2. (Relates to data)
3. (1) d
   (2) a
   (3) f
   (4) c
   (5) b
   (6) e

4. Hyperkalemia may cause the production of ectopic pacemakers and result in fibrillation. These effects are produced because a rise in plasma potassium concentrations depolarizes the cell membrane and thus makes the myocardial cells hyperexcitable.

5. Adding Ca^{++} increased the amplitude of the heart's contraction. The heartbeat was stronger, but relaxation was less complete. This occurred because Ca^{++} stimulates muscle contraction by allowing formation of myosin cross-bridges, so more cross-bridges were formed. Relaxation decreases because it is difficult to remove all of the Ca^{++} from the muscle cell.
6. Digitalis causes the heart to beat more strongly and it decreases the rate of impulse conduction from the atria to the ventricles. The latter effect makes the ventricles beat more slowly. As a result of these actions, digitalis may be used in congestive heart failure to increase the pumping strength of the heart, and it may be used to treat atrial flutter and fibrillation by decreasing the rate of beat of the ventricles.

Laboratory Report 33 Electrocardiogram

A. Electrocardiogram at Rest

1. (Relates to data)
2. SA node
3. a. depolarization of the atria
   b. depolarization of the ventricles
   c. repolarization of the ventricles
4. extrasystole
5. first-degree AV node block
6. ventricular fibrillation
7. The SA node undergoes spontaneous depolarization after its action potential is completed. As a result, it produces action potentials that are conducted to other cells that have the capacity for spontaneous depolarization but have slower cycles than the cells of the SA node. All of the cells stimulated by action potentials that originated in the SA node contract at the same time and thus are paced by the SA node.
8. In paroxysmal supraventricular tachycardia, the atria beat rapidly for periods of time and, as a result of the conduction of impulses into the ventricles, cause the ventricles to beat rapidly. The ECG is rapid but normal in appearance, and the ventricles are able to pump blood during this condition. In ventricular tachycardia, the ventricles are not paced by the atria but rather by ectopic foci in the ventricles, which cause the ECG to have a saw-toothed appearance. This condition is very serious because it can degenerate into ventricular fibrillation, and because ventricular pumping is very erratic.
9. At the time of the initial examination, the patient had first-degree AV node block. A year later it appears that the damage to the AV node has become more severe. The person now has third-degree AV node block because an ectopic pacemaker appears in the ventricles, which results in a very slow rate of beat.

B. Electrocardiogram following Exercise

1. (Relates to data)
2. QRS
3. T
4. P
5. At the beginning of exercise, there is a decrease in the activity of the vagus innervation of the heart. This causes an increase in cardiac rate, which is further stimulated at greater levels of exercise by increased sympathetic nerve activity. As a result of the faster rate, the period of diastole is shortened, so that the time between the T wave of one ECG pattern and the P wave of the next is significantly reduced.

6. At rest, the delivery of blood to the heart may be adequate for the needs of the myocardium despite the possibility that there may be some occlusion of the coronary blood flow. After moderate exercise, the myocardial demand for oxygen is raised, so that the myocardium may become ischemic as a result of the coronary occlusion. This myocardial ischemia may thus be revealed in the ECG taken during exercise but not in the resting ECG pattern.

Laboratory Report 34 Mean Electrical Axis of the Ventricles

1. (Relates to data)
2. (Relates to data)
3. (Relates to data)
4. The spread of action potentials into the ventricles produces the QRS wave. As the impulses spread out from the interventricular septum into the myocardium and one region of the ventricles is depolarized while other regions are not, a potential difference is created in the ventricles. This potential difference is seen by an upward deflection of the ECG from the baseline (Q to R). When the entire mass of the ventricles is depolarized, all regions have the same polarity. Since at this time there is no potential difference in the ventricles, the ECG pattern returns to the baseline (R to S).
5. If there is a block in a branch of the interventricular bundle, it will take longer for action potentials to travel into the region of the ventricles served by that branch. A block in the left branch, for example, will cause the left ventricle to be depolarized more slowly than the right. Similarly, if one ventricle is hypertrophied, a longer time will be required to depolarize the thicker muscle of that ventricle. Whenever added time is needed to depolarize one ventricle, the mean electrical axis will deviate in the direction of that ventricle.

Laboratory Report 35 Heart Sounds and Measurement of Blood Pressure

A. Heart Sounds

1. Since the heart valves do not conduct action potentials, they do not affect the ECG patterns. Structural defects in the valves may affect the pattern of blood flow in the heart, however, and abnormal patterns of blood flow can cause abnormal vibrations and thus abnormal heart sounds, which can be heard by auscultation.
2. Splitting of the heart sounds refers to hearing two separate components to the lub (first sound) and/or the dub (second sound). This is caused by separate closure of the two AV valves or separate closure of the aortic and pulmonary valves.
3. The QRS wave represents ventricular depolarization. When the ventricles depolarize, they are stimulated to contract, which causes the AV valves to close and produce the first heart sound. The T wave represents ventricular repolarization. When the ventricles repolarize, they begin to relax, which causes the semilunar valves to close and produce the second heart sound.

B. Measurement of Blood Pressure

1. (Relates to data)
2. systolic pressure, diastolic pressure
3. a. 165
   b. 110
   c. 55
   d. 128

4. The person has hypertension. This is dangerous because of increased susceptibility to atherosclerosis, heart disease, and stroke.
5. The sounds of Korotkoff are caused by the vibrations produced by the turbulent flow of blood in an artery. Normally, blood flows in a laminar pattern and the absence of turbulence causes the blood flow to be silent. When the pressure cuff partially constricts the artery, the narrowing of the lumen creates turbulence and the Korotkoff sounds.
6. The position of the arm directly affects the measurement of diastolic pressure because of the effect of gravity. When the arm is below heart level, the diastolic pressure is raised, and when it is above heart level, the diastolic pressure is lowered.

Laboratory Report 36 Cardiovascular System and Physical Fitness

1. (Relates to data)
2. Yes, a person's aerobic capacity decreases with age beyond about age 29. This results in part from the fact that the maximum cardiac rate decreases with age, accompanied by a decrease in cardiac output and thus in the maximal rate of oxygen delivery to the tissues.
3. A person who is physically fit may have a higher stroke volume and cardiac output, which increases the rate of blood flow. Also, the muscles have an increased ability to extract oxygen from the blood because of biochemical changes within the muscle cells.
4. A person who is physically fit requires less of an increase in cardiac output for a given level of exercise. The blood pressure and pulse rate thus do not increase as much as in a person who is not physically fit.
5. The heart has only a limited ability to respire anaerobically, and thus if oxygen delivery is inadequate for an extended period, myocardial ischemia and infarction may occur. Since exercise raises the myocardial demand for oxygen, the presence of myocardial ischemia, with consequent changes in the ECG, may be evident after exercise but not at rest. This could be caused by a coronary thrombosis that partially occludes a coronary artery.

Laboratory Report 37 Respiratory System

1. The primary function of the respiratory system is to transport gases to and from the alveoli of the lungs. The basic functional unit of the respiratory system is the alveoli.
2. The advantages of breathing through your nose instead of your mouth are (1) the nasal epithelia covering the conchae warm, moisten, and cleanse the air and (2) olfactory epithelia in the upper posterior portion of the nasal cavity are associated with the olfactory reception of odors.
3. The transport of gases to and from the tissues of the body depends upon a close relationship between the respiratory system and the circulatory system. Oxygen is taken into the body via the respiratory system and is transferred to the circulatory system via the alveoli-capillary junction. It is then transported to the tissues of the body. Carbon dioxide leaves the tissues of the body and enters the circulatory system. Finally, the carbon dioxide leaves the circulatory system and enters the alveoli of the lungs. This gas is exhaled from the body.
4. The nasopharynx serves only the respiratory system as it receives inspired air from the nasal cavity. It contains the pharyngeal tonsils and the opening of the auditory tube. The oropharynx serves the respiratory and digestive systems. It contains the palatine and lingual tonsils. The laryngopharynx is superior to the larynx and serves the respiratory and digestive systems. It opens inferiorly into the glottis and the esophagus.
5. Cartilage elements in the larynx, trachea, and bronchi provide flexibility and support to the structures, so that air passageways are always open.
6. Refer to figure 37.2 in the *Laboratory Manual.* Food and water are supposed to pass into the esophagus, but occasionally the epiglottis doesn't close and food or water enters the trachea—the wrong pipe.

7. Infections and diseases are effectively blocked from spreading from one pleural cavity to the other. Furthermore, a pneumothorax (air entering one pleural cavity) will cause one lung to collapse but not the other lung.
8. The left lung has a cardiac notch and is subdivided into superior and inferior lobes. The right lung is subdivided into superior, middle, and inferior lobes. Each lung is covered by a visceral pleura and is situated in its own pleural space. Each lung has a mediastinal surface where the pulmonary vessels traverse, a base contacting the diaphragm, a costal surface contacting the rib cage, and an apex pointing superiorly.

Laboratory Report 38 Measurements of Pulmonary Function

A. Measurement of Simple Lung Volumes and Capacities

1. (Relates to data)

B. Measurement of Forced Expiratory Volume

1. (Relates to data)
2. (Relates to data)
3. a. vital capacity 4500 cc
   b. inspiratory reserve volume 3000 cc
   c. inspiratory capacity 3500 cc
   d. residual volume 1500 cc
4. a. 800 cc
   b. 3100 cc
   c. 1450 cc
   d. 4550 cc
5. 77.3%
6. obstructive
7. asthma
8. $FEV_{1.0}$ test
9. Your lungs inflate because your chest expands. Contraction of the diaphragm and intercostal muscles increases the volume of the thorax and lungs. This increased volume creates a subatmospheric pressure; as a result, air is pushed into the lungs.
10. Obstructive disease is present when there is an abnormally high resistance to airflow through the bronchioles due to bronchoconstriction or mucus. In obstructive disorders, vital capacity is normal, but $FEV_{1.0}$ is low. Restrictive disorders occur when the alveoli are affected by disease. Thus vital capacity is reduced, but $FEV_{1.0}$ is normal. Spirometry is useful in the diagnosis of lung diseases. On the basis of pulmonary function tests, lung disorders can be classified as obstructive or restrictive. In restrictive disorders, vital capacity is reduced to a level below normal. In obstructive disorders, the rate of expiration is decreased.

Laboratory Report 39 Effects of Exercise on the Respiratory System

A. Total Minute Volume and Oxygen Consumption

1. (Relates to data)
2. (Relates to data)

3. During exercise, the rate of metabolism of the exercising muscles increased, so they consumed oxygen at an increased rate. Immediately after exercise, the rate of oxygen consumption remained elevated as a result of the increased need for oxygen in metabolizing the lactic acid and the increased amount of oxygen consumed by the muscles warmed during exercise.
4. The total minute volume increased during exercise and remained high immediately after exercise. The increase in total minute volume during exercise may be due to chemoreceptor stimulation and to neural reflexes involving the exercising muscles. The continued high total minute volume after exercising is produced through chemoreceptor stimulation by the increased production of carbon dioxide by the muscles.
5. In hyperpnea, the high total minute volume produced during exercise is matched by a high rate of metabolism. As a result, the rate at which carbon dioxide is produced by the tissues is matched by the rate at which it is "blown off" and arterial CO_2 concentrations are normal. During hyperventilation, in contrast, blood CO_2 concentrations fall.
6. The term oxygen debt refers to the increased amount of oxygen consumed by the body after exercise has ceased. This is required to metabolize the lactic acid produced during exercise and to support the increased metabolism of the muscles warmed during exercise. Hyperpnea continues for a time after exercise has stopped so that the oxygen debt incurred during exercise can be repaid. The rate of oxygen uptake slowly returns to normal so that oxygen levels can be restored to normal.

B. Effect of Exercise on the Rate of CO_2 Production

1. (Relates to data)
2. (Relates to data)
3. a. An acid donates protons (H^+) to solution.
   b. A base removes protons from solution, usually by releasing OH^-, which combines with H^+ to form H_2CO_3.
   c. Acidosis is the condition in which the blood pH is less than 7.35.
   d. Alkalosis is the condition in which the blood pH is greater than 7.45.
4. 9; 10^{-5}M
5. acidosis, alkalosis
6. hypoventilation: increased CO_2 drives the following equation to the right:
   $CO_2 + H_2O \rightleftharpoons H_2CO_3 \rightleftharpoons H^+ + HCO_3^-$
   Therefore, the concentration of both H^+ and HCO_3^- will rise.
7. A rise in the blood bicarbonate levels produced by the intravenous infusion combines with and buffers the free H^+, which is causing the acidosis: $HCO_3^- + H^+ \rightleftharpoons H_2CO_3$.

Laboratory Report 40 Urinary System

1. Refer to figure 40.2 in the lab manual.
2. The kidneys are retroperitoneal and lie on each side of the vertebral column high in the abdominal cavity from the level of the twelfth thoracic to the third lumbar vertebra. The right kidney is usually 1.5–2.0 cm lower than the left kidney because of the large area occupied by the liver.
3. a. glomeruli, glomerular (Bowman's) capsule, proximal convoluted tubule, distal convoluted tubule
   b. nephron loop (loop of Henle), collecting duct
4. interlobular artery, afferent arteriole, glomerulus, efferent arteriole, peritubular capillaries, interlobular vein
5. glomerular (Bowman's) capsule, proximal convoluted tubule, descending limb, nephron loop (loop of Henle), ascending limb, distal convoluted tubule, collecting duct, renal calyx, renal pelvis, ureter, urinary bladder, urethra

Laboratory Report 41 Renal Regulation of Fluid and Electrolyte Balance

1. (Relates to data)
2. antidiuretic hormone (ADH)
3. aldosterone
4. 5 mEq/L of Ca^{++}
5.

	Prospector	*Party goer*
urine volume	lower	higher
specific gravity	higher	lower
Na^+, Cl^-	lower	higher

6. The desert prospector probably has a higher secretion of ADH because he is more dehydrated than the party goer. The party goer has become overly hydrated and has drunk alcohol, which inhibits ADH secretion. The party goer would therefore excrete a larger volume of more dilute urine than the prospector. This more dilute urine would have a lower specific gravity. Since the prospector may be dehydrated, he may have a higher secretion of aldosterone than the party goer. In this case, aldosterone would stimulate increased reabsorption of Na^+ and Cl^-, so that less is excreted in the urine.
7. Drugs that inhibit the reabsorption of Na^+ in the nephron loop cause an increased urinary excretion of Na^+ and also of Cl^- because Cl^- follows the Na^+ passively. Increased excretion of K^+ also occurs, as a result of the increased secretion of K^+ into the filtrate by the distal tubule. This results from the fact that, as a consequence of the diuretic drug, the exchange of Na^+ for K^+ in the distal tubule occurs at a faster rate.

Laboratory Report 42 Renal Plasma Clearance of Urea

1. (Relates to data)
2. (Relates to data)
3. (Relates to data)
4. (Relates to data)
5. a. inulin
   b. urea
   c. PAH
   d. creatinine
   e. protein
6. a. urea
   b. inulin
   c. creatinine
   d. PAH
7. The renal plasma clearance rate (ml/min) of a given compound is the milliliters of plasma that originally contained the amount of that compound excreted per minute in the urine. The clearance rate is measured by obtaining the excretion rate of a compound (mg/min) and dividing that figure by the concentration of that compound (mg/ml) in the blood.
8. a. Increased catabolism of proteins liberates increased amounts of amino acids that can be deaminated, thus increasing the amount of amine groups that can be used to form urea.
   b. Decreased blood pressure can decrease the glomerular filtration rate, so that the excretion of urea is reduced and the concentration of urea in the blood is consequently increased.
   c. If the kidneys fail to produce urine, the concentration of urea in the blood will increase because urea will still be continuously formed but not excreted.

Laboratory Report 43 Clinical Examination of the Urine

1. (Relates to data)
2. a. diabetes mellitus
   b. glomerular inflammation
   c. weight loss, fasting
   d. liver disease or bile duct obstruction
3. Casts are composed of proteins that have leaked through inflamed glomeruli, which have become more permeable to proteins as a result of the inflammation.
4. Yes. The person may have hyperglycemia, but the blood glucose concentration may be below the renal plasma threshold for glucose.
5. If kidney disease causes the abnormal excretion of plasma proteins in the urine, the concentration of plasma protein will be reduced. As a result, the colloid osmotic pressure of the plasma will be decreased. This prevents the normal return of tissue fluid to the blood and results in edema.

Laboratory Report 44 Digestive System

A. Organization of the Digestive System

1. oral cavity, pharynx, esophagus, stomach, duodenum, jejunum, ileum, cecum, ascending colon, transverse colon, descending colon, sigmoid colon, rectum, and anal canal
2. The mucosa consists of lining epithelium, connective tissue of the lamina propria, and smooth muscle of the muscularis mucosa.
   The submucosa consists of connective tissue.
   The muscularis externa consists of longitudinal and circular layers of smooth muscle.
   The serosa consists of loose connective tissue.

B. Serous Membranes of the Gastrointestinal Tract

1. The lesser omentum is a connective tissue membrane joining the lesser curvature of the stomach to the liver.
2. The greater omentum is an apronlike connective tissue membrane with abundant adipose tissue extending from the greater curvature of the stomach to the level of the transverse colon.
3. Mesenteries are connective tissue membranes extending between the loops of the small intestine and from the dorsal body wall to the gastrointestinal tract.

C. Mouth, Pharynx, and Associated Structures

1. The stratified squamous membrane offers protection against abrasion and desiccation.
2. During swallowing, a bolus is formed as the tongue is elevated against the palate through contraction of the mylohyoid and styloglossus muscles and the intrinsic muscles of the tongue. Pressure of the tongue against the rugae of the hard palate seals the pharynx from the oral cavity, creates pressure, and forces the bolus into the pharynx. The elevation of the larynx against the epiglottis seals the glottis so that food or liquid is less likely to enter the trachea.

D. Esophagus and Stomach

1. The mucosa of the esophagus is stratified squamous to afford protection against abrasion and desiccation. The muscularis of the esophagus is composed of striated muscle in the superior region of the esophagus to aid voluntary control of swallowing. The mucosa of the stomach consists of a simple columnar epithelium for secretion and limited absorption. The muscularis of the stomach is composed of three layers of smooth muscle for the churning actions required.
2. a. The gastric rugae are folds of submucosa and mucosa in the stomach.
   b. The gastric glands are simple tubular glands formed by invagination of the gastric mucosa. These glands secrete HCl and pepsinogen.

E and F. Small Intestine and Large Intestine

1. Villi are fingerlike projections of mucosa in the small intestine. They are covered by a simple columnar epithelium, with the epithelial cell membranes folded to form microvilli on the luminal side. The villi and microvilli provide a high surface area for absorption of digestion products. Amino acids and monosaccharides are absorbed into blood capillaries within the lamina propria core of the villus. Absorbed fat is absorbed into the central lacteal, which is a lymphatic capillary within the villus.
2. a. Plicae circulares are folds of submucosa in the small intestine.
   b. The ileum is the longest region of the small intestine.
   c. The cecum is a pouch at the beginning of the large intestine, into which the ileum empties.
   d. The haustra are pouchlike structures seen on the surface of the large intestine.
   e. Taenia coli are bands of smooth muscle that are visible on the surface of the large intestine.

G. Liver, Gallbladder, and Pancreas

1. Liver lobules are microscopic organizations of liver tissue. Each lobule consists of many hepatic plates separated by blood sinusoids that drain into a central vein. At the periphery of each lobule are a number of portal triads. Each triad consists of a branch of the hepatic portal vein, hepatic artery, and bile duct.
2. Blood flows from the portal triads, through the sinusoids, and into the central vein of the liver lobule. Bile flows in bile canaliculi within hepatic plates, from the central regions of the lobule to the hepatic ducts within the portal triads. In this way, blood and bile are kept separate within the liver.
3. The hepatic duct drains bile out of the liver. The cystic duct carries bile to the gallbladder.
4. The pancreas contains exocrine acini, which are clusters of cells that produce pancreatic juice and secrete this exocrine product into branches of the pancreatic duct. Scattered within the exocrine acini are encapsulated islands of endocrine tissue, the pancreatic islets, which produce insulin and glucagon and secrete these hormones into blood capillaries.

Laboratory Report 45 Digestion of Starch by Salivary Amylase

1. (Relates to data)
2. Following incubation, tubes 1 and 4 contained the most starch, and tube 2 contained the most sugar. One can conclude that salivary amylase functions best at a neutral pH and is at least partially destroyed by boiling.
3. If the tests for both starch and sugar are positive at the end of the incubation, one can conclude that the starch was partially digested. If the incubation had proceeded for a longer time, eventually the test for starch would be negative, since all of the starch would be digested.
4. Once salivary amylase reached the gastric juice in the stomach, it would be inactivated. This is shown by tube 3, in which the addition of HCl inhibited the action of this enzyme.

5. Cooking reduces or completely abolishes enzyme activity. This occurs because enzymes are denatured by heat (their tertiary structure is destroyed).

Laboratory Report 46 Digestion of Egg Albumin by Pepsin

1. (Relates to data)
2. The most digestion occurred in tube 2. This shows that pepsin has an acidic pH optimum.
3. Hydrochloric acid stimulated the digestive action of pepsin, whereas it inhibited the digestive action of salivary amylase. This is because of the different pH optima of these two enzymes. Pepsin is adapted to work in the acidic environment of gastric juice, whereas salivary amylase is adapted to work at the nearly neutral pH of saliva.
4. As shown in tube 5, freezing inhibits the action of enzymes. Food that is frozen keeps longer because the enzymes in organisms that promote decomposition (bacteria and fungi) are inhibited under these conditions.
5. The stomach doesn't normally digest itself because of the protective effects of mucus, the tight junctions between adjacent epithelial cells, and the rapid rate of cell division, which acts to replace damaged epithelial cells. Gastric juice does not normally digest the duodenum because the acidic gastric juice is rapidly neutralized by the arrival of alkaline pancreatic juice.

Laboratory Report 47 Digestion of Fat by Pancreatic Juice and Bile

1. (Relates to data)
2. As triglycerides (fat) undergo hydrolysis reactions during digestion, free fatty acids are liberated from the neutral triglyceride molecules. These free fatty acids lower the pH of the solution.
3. Bile lowers the surface tension around globules of fat and in this way breaks up larger fat globules into smaller globules. Since these smaller globules still contain triglyceride molecules—that is, since no hydrolysis reactions have occurred in the process of emulsification—digestion cannot be said to have occurred.
4. Fat digestion occurred most rapidly in tube 3. This is because the fat emulsified by bile presented the largest surface area for digestion by the lipase enzymes. Digestion occurred more slowly in tube 2 because the fat was not emulsified and thus presented a smaller surface area for digestion by lipase. Digestion did not occur at all in tube 1 because this tube did not contain lipase.
5. If the excretion of bile is blocked by gallstones, bilirubin will accumulate in the blood because it cannot be excreted in the bile. This can result in jaundice. If the secretion of bile into the intestine is blocked, fat digestion and absorption will be impaired. This could reduce the absorption of fat-soluble vitamins, including vitamin K. If the person is deficient in vitamin K, the ability to form the clotting factors will be impaired, thus accounting for the prolonged clotting time.
6. Once fatty acids and monoglycerides enter the intestinal epithelial cells, they are used to resynthesize triglycerides. These triglycerides are then secreted into the central lacteals and enter the lymphatic drainage. Glucose and amino acids, in contrast, are absorbed through the intestinal epithelial cells without being changed and are then secreted directly into the blood.

Laboratory Report 48 Caloric Balance and Body Weight

Three-Day Dietary Records

(Relates to data)

Three-Day Dietary Record Evaluation

(Relates to data)

General Questions

1. Since one pound of fat is equivalent to 3,500 kilocalories, 20 pounds of fat are equivalent to 70,000 kilocalories. This is 7,000 kilocalories per month for 10 months. Dividing 7,000 kilocalories per month by 4 weeks per month gives 1,750 kilocalories per week. The student must thus eat 1,750 kilocalories per week less than is consumed by metabolism to lose 20 pounds by graduation.
2. Dividing 1,750 kilocalories per week by 7 days per week gives 250 kilocalories per day. This is certainly a practical weight loss program, as 250 kilocalories per day might be saved by merely substituting low-fat food for their equivalents (e.g., baked potato instead of french fries, etc.).
3. Dividing 250 kilocalories per day by 9 kilocalories per gram of fat gives about 28 g of fat. This amount of fat could be removed from the diet in many cases. (In practical terms, however, some fat will be present in the food.)
4. The basal metabolic rate (BMR) is the metabolic rate under resting conditions, 12 hours after eating, and in a comfortable environment. Physical activity usually raises the total energy consumption by at least 30%.

Laboratory Report 49 Reproductive System

A. Male Reproductive System

1. seminiferous tubules, rete testis, efferent ductules, head of the epididymis, tail of the epididymis, ductus (vas) deferens, ejaculatory duct, prostatic urethra, membranous urethra, spongy urethra
2. In a vasectomy, the ductus (vas) deferens is cut and tied. This interferes with the transport of sperm to the ejaculatory duct but does not affect the secretion of testosterone. This is because testosterone is a hormone secreted into the blood by the interstitial cells.
3. The descent of the testes begins between the sixth and tenth week. Descent into the scrotal sac, however, does not occur until about the twenty-eighth week, when paired inguinal canals form in the abdominal wall. The descent of a testis appears to depend on the shortening of the gubernaculum, which is attached to the testis and extends through the inguinal canal to the scrotum. As the testis descends, it carries with it the ductus (vas) deferens, the testicular vessels and nerve, a portion of the abdominal muscle, and lymph vessels. These structures remain attached to the testis and become the spermatic cord.

B. Female Reproductive System

1. The clitoris is homologous to the glans penis, and the labia majora are homologous to the scrotum.
2. The superficial layer of the endometrium, called the stratum functionale, is shed during menstruation. This layer is developed from the underlying stratum basale during the weeks prior to menstruation. The myometrium contains smooth muscle, which is required for labor and delivery. The myometrium also contains elastic tissue that allows the uterus to stretch to accommodate the growing fetus. The perimetrium is composed of connective tissue.

3. The ovarian follicles grow prior to ovulation. One of these, the graafian follicle, continues to grow and ovulate. After ovulation, the empty follicle becomes a corpus luteum, which degenerates just prior to menstruation.

Laboratory Report 50 Steroid Hormones

1. (Relates to data)
2. estradiol; testosterone
3. a. estradiol
   b. testosterone
   c. progesterone
4. corpus luteum; placenta
5. aldosterone; hydrocortisone
6. Testosterone and deoxycorticosterone have the highest R_f values and therefore are the most soluble in the solvent. The glucocorticoids (corticosterone, hydrocortisone, and cortisone) have the lowest R_f values and thus are the least soluble. Estradiol is intermediate between these extremes.
7. Refer to figures 19.10 and 19.11 in *Concepts of Human Anatomy and Physiology,* 4th edition. Mineralocorticoids are produced in the adrenal cortex. Glucocorticoids are produced in the adrenal cortex. Sex steroids are produced in the adrenal cortex, ovaries, and testes.

Laboratory Report 51 Pregnancy Test

1. corpus luteum
2. trophoblast cells of the blastocyst
3. luteinizing hormone (LH)
4. The corpus luteum is formed from the empty ovulated follicle under stimulation by LH. Once formed, the corpus luteum secretes estradiol and progesterone during the luteal phase of the cycle. The estradiol and progesterone during the luteal phase exert negative feedback inhibition of gonadotropin secretion from the anterior pituitary, and as a consequence of the low LH that results, the corpus luteum dies at the end of a nonfertile cycle. When fertilization occurs, the embryo secretes hCG, which acts like LH on the corpus luteum and maintains it for the first ten weeks of pregnancy.
5. Although hCG is secreted in small amounts very shortly after conception, the levels of hCG must rise high enough to be within the sensitivity of the pregnancy test in order for that test to be valid.
6. It is called an immunoassay because it is based on the combination of antibodies against hCG with hCG antigens. In the test performed, particles of latex rubber were coated with these antibodies and mixed with samples of urine. If the urine contained hCG, the combination of hCG with the antibodies caused the particles of latex rubber to agglutinate.

Laboratory Report 52 Patterns of Heredity

A. Sickle-Cell Anemia

(Relates to data)

B. Inheritance of PTC Taste

(Relates to data)

C. Sex-Linked Traits: Inheritance of Color Blindness

(Relates to data)

General Questions

1. If T = taster and t = nontaster, the father is *tt*, the student is *Tt*, and the mother is either *TT* or *Tt*.
2. a. 50%
   b. 50%
3. The probability that their first child will have hemophilia is 25%; this is the same for the next child because the probability for each event is independent of the other events. The sex of the child is male. This is because hemophilia is inherited on the X chromosome and the male always gets his X chromosome from his mother (who in this case is a carrier for hemophilia). Females get one X chromosome from their mother and one from their father, who carries only the dominant normal gene.

Appendix A Biological Supply Houses

Aloe Scientific Company
5655 Kingsburg
St. Louis, MO 63112

Baltimore Biological Lab., Inc.
1640 Grosuch Avenue
Baltimore, MD 21204

Bico Scientific Company
2325 South Michigan Avenue
Chicago, IL 60616

Biocom, Inc.
9522 West Jefferson Boulevard
Culver City, CA 90230

Calbiochem
10933 North Torrey Pines Road
La Jolla, CA 92037

Carolina Biological Supply Co.
2700 York Road
Burlington, NC 27215

Central Scientific Company
2600 South Kostner Avenue
Chicago, IL 60623

Clay-Adams Company
141 East Twenty-fifth Street
New York, NY 10037

College Biological Supply Company
Box 25017 Northgate Station
Seattle, WA 98125

Denoyer-Geppert Company
5235 Ravenswood Avenue
Chicago, IL 60640

E & M Instrument Company, Inc.
150 Endicott Street
Norwood, MA 02062

Faust Scientific Supply Co.
Madison, WI 53713

Fisher Scientific Company
1232 North Honore Street
Chicago, IL 60622

Gilson Medical Electronics
3000 West Beltline Highway
Middleton, WI 53562

Harvard Apparatus Co., Inc.
150 Dover Road
Millis, MA 02054

Lapine Scientific Company
6001 South Knox Avenue
Chicago, IL 60629

Macalaster Scientific Corp.
Waltham Research and Developmental Park
186 Third Avenue
Waltham, MA 02154

Matheson Scientific Company
2909 Highland Avenue
Norwood, OH 45212

Medical Plastics Laboratory
P.O. Box 38
Gatesville, TX 76528

Merck and Company, Inc.
Rahway, NJ 07065

Narco Bio-Systems, Inc.
7651 Airport Boulevard
Houston, TX 77017

Nasco, Inc.
Fort Atkinson, WI 53538

Phipps and Bird, Inc.
303 South Sixth Street
Richmond, VA 23205

Sargent-Welch Scientific Co.
7300 North Linder Avenue
Skokie, IL 60078

Scientific Products
1210 Waukegan Road
McGraw Park, IL 60085

Turtox/Cambosco
Macmillan Science Company
8200 Hoyne Avenue
Chicago, IL 60620

Van Waters and Rogers
1363 South Bonnie Beach Place
Los Angeles, CA 90023

Ward's Natural Science Establishment, Inc.
P.O. Box 1712
Rochester, NY 14603

West Coast Scientific Company
P.O. Box 2947
Oakland, CA 94618

Appendix B Commonly Used Solutions

Benedict's Reagent

1. Dissolve 50 g sodium carbonate, 85.0 g sodium citrate, and 8.5 g copper sulfate in 5.0 liters of water.

Biuret Reagent

1. Add 45 g of sodium potassium tartate and 15 g of $CuSO_4{-}5H_2O$ to a 1.0-liter volumetric flask.
2. Fill the flask three-quarters full with 0.2*N* NaOH and shake to dissolve.
3. Add 5.0 g of potassium iodide, and fill to volume with 0.2*N* NaOH.

Developing Solvent for Thin-layer Chromatography

1. The developing solvent should be mixed in a 6:1:1 volume ratio of benzene, ethyl acetate, and acetone in whatever volume is appropriate for your class size.

Ringer's Solution

1. Dissolve 6 g NaCl, 0.075 g KCl, 0.10 g $CaCl_2$, and 0.10 g $NaHCO_3$ in 1.0 liter of water.

Other solutions used in the lab are mixed to molar, molal, normal, or g% concentrations, and those concentrations are listed in the exercises themselves.

Appendix C Tips on Dissection

Dissection can be a time-consuming and tedious process. However, there is no greater tool in learning anatomy than a well-dissected cadaver. For this reason, we wish to give a few general instructions that may aid in performing a dissection. Perhaps the most important concept in dissection is care for the specimen, and for the dissection itself. This involves two things: maintenance of the cadavers, and performing a thoughtful dissection.

Cadavers must be kept moist at all times. Exposed areas should be wet frequently, and areas that are not being studied should be kept covered with moist towels. A wetting solution should be used to keep the cadavers moist. Wetting solution is typically made of a mixture of pheonol, propylene glycol, and water, but the method of preparation of the cadaver will dictate what solution should be used. Particular attention must be paid to keeping the head, hands, feet, and genitalia moist, since these areas tend to dry out quickly. Covering the head, hands, and feet with plastic bags over the moist toweling will help prevent desiccation of the specimens. If the cadavers are not kept moist, they will dry out, and the muscles stiffen and lose their color.

A dissection must be performed with thought and planning. Be aware of which structures will be encountered during the dissection, and the order in which they will be encountered. Be aware of surface landmarks and bony processes that may be usedful in locating internal structures. Be aware of the fragility or durability of specific structures or organs you encounter, so you can take precautions to protect the specimen. Dissect with a plan instead of mindlessly searching for one structure while destroying other important structures.

Materials Needed for Dissection

1. *Atlas*. A good atlas is essential to show the structures you are dissecting. Atlases will also provide views from different perspectives of the cadaver to add to the learning experience.
2. *Forceps (2 pair)*. A large pair and small pair of forceps should be available to use in holding structures and in removing fatty tissue.
3. *Scissors (2 pair)*. A large pair and small pair of scissors should be available.
4. *Probe*. A probe can be useful for performing blunt dissection as well as for holding structures out of the way.
5. *Scalpel*. A scalpel is very useful in dissection, but it must be used with care. Scalpels are very sharp and therefore can make deep cuts into the cadaver or specimen. They also have potential to injure the dissector if not used carefully. Make sure you have a proper container for disposal of used scalpel blades.
6. *Wetting solution*. The cadaver must be kept moist at all times, especially during dissection.

Specific Hints for Dissection

1. Keep your instruments sharp at all times.
2. When removing the skin, remove only the skin. Many veins and some muscles are located very close to the skin in the subcutaneous fat and can be dissected away if careful attention is not paid. Therefore, care must be taken to remove as little fat as possible if you wish to preserve these superficial structures. After making an incision in the skin, place tension on the skin by pulling it away from the body in order to separate the skin from the subcutaneous fat.
3. Be careful when removing fat from around structures. Many structures are embedded in fat, and glandular tissue bears a striking resemblence to fatty tissue, especially to the untrained eye. Organs that pose particular problems are the pancreas, adrenal glands, parotid and submandibular glands, and inguinal and axillary lymph nodes.
4. When superficial muscles must be removed to expose deep structures, the muscle should be detached at either its origin or its insertion, instead of cutting it through the middle of the muscle belly.

5. In order to view the structures of the thoracic cavity, the rib cage must be removed. Once the superficial muscles are separated, the rib cage may be removed in two ways. The top of the rib cage may be removed by cutting through the manubrium with a bone saw or cutting the clavicle near the acromioclavicular joint. Either method will allow adequate access to the thoracic cavity. Removal of the clavicles will allow for viewing of the vessels which come off the aortic arch, as well as the subclavian vessels. After the top of the rib cage is cut, the ribs must then be cut down the sides with the bone saw. Be careful using the bone saw because bone chips may be projected from the saw, and the edges of the bone may be very sharp. The diaphragm must be carefully removed from the rib cage. This is most easily accomplished from the inside of the thoracic cavity.
6. Arteries and veins may be separated from one another by carefully inserting a closed pair of scissors between the two, and then opening the scissors along the longitudinal axis of the vessels. This will create a small separation which can then be bluntly dissected with the fingers to separate the vessels. Take particular care with arteries, veins, and nerves because they are particularly fragile.